Rural Health

Rural Health

A FRAMEWORK FOR UNDERSTANDING THE ISSUES AND THEIR IMPACT ON RURAL POPULATIONS

First Edition

Maria C. Clay and Rebecca W. Lewis

East Carolina University

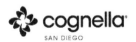
cognella®
SAN DIEGO

Bassim Hamadeh, CEO and Publisher
Susana Christie, Senior Developmental Editor
Anne Jones, Project Editor
Abbey Hastings, Production Editor
Asfa Arshi, Graphic Design Assistant
Trey Soto, Licensing Specialist
Jaye Pratt, Interior Designer
Natalie Piccotti, Director of Marketing
Kassie Graves, Senior Vice President of Editorial
Jamie Giganti, Director of Academic Publishing

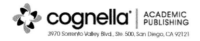

3970 Sorrento Valley Blvd., Ste. 500, San Diego, CA 92121

Contents

Preface

When rural health is taught, practiced, or researched, the approach is often on what is missing or lacking in terms of health care resources, health care access, and preferred health outcomes. While it is accepted that rural health is unique and complex, there are few conceptual models or theories to guide us. Instead, professionals from various disciplines and educational backgrounds who gather data and analyze the health disparities of rural populations and plan appropriate interventions may not be guided by a unifying framework or theory. However, the complexity of rural health and the interprofessional nature of rural health solutions creates the need for a rural health framework that will systematically examine and direct the planning of health care interventions. The Rural Health Framework fulfills that need.

The Rural Health Framework evolved from a 2005 undergraduate course taught by Dr. Maria Clay and Dr. Annette Greer. In 2011, Rebecca Lewis became the third course instructor. (The running case in Chapter 1 is a fuller description of the historical context and development of the Rural Health Framework.) Each semester that the course was taught, the content improved, based upon student feedback and thoughtful instructor reflection. Today the course is a vital part of the educational preparation for many of the health sciences disciplines, including public health, pharmacy dentistry, medicine, nursing, physical therapy, nutrition, and social work. The Rural Health Framework, then, is a result of a collaboration of faculty, students, and practitioners who used the framework to understand and guide rural health.

Acknowledgments

Acknowledgment for both the development of the Rural Health Framework and many of the design features for our teaching of the Framework must first and foremost go to Dr. Annette Greer. As a student, on-site coordinator, and eventually co-director of the Interdisciplinary Rural Health Education Office, Dr. Greer was instrumental in designing the coursework that comprises the Interdisciplinary Rural Health Education at both the undergraduate and graduate level. Her knowledge of and commitment to health in rural areas informs many of the issues and content of the IRHE course upon which this book is based.

Second, we owe a tremendous appreciation to the vision of Dr. Doyle "Skip" Cummings, the Co-PI of the Quentin Burdick Rural Health Training Program Grant, which took us into the community and began our journey into understanding rural health and the issues that impact health for rural communities.

Drs. Bonita Sasnett and Patricia Royal, two of our on-site coordinators, spent years understanding the needs of university students in the rural communities and developing meaningful programs to help interprofessional students know one another and appreciate the nuances of rural health. Mr. Emanual Hyman later joined Drs. Sasnett and Royal, contributing his own unique skill set to the teaching of Rural Health while Dr. Sheila Simmons focused on campus courses and student needs.

We are deeply grateful to the thousands of students who have taken our courses, expanded our vision of what rural health should and could be, and taught us the importance of a clearly defined framework upon which to anchor learning.

We are also grateful for the guidance and flexibility of our editorial staff at Cognella. When we started the book, we did not imagine completing it during a pandemic that would underscore the very issues highlighted in the Framework but which also presented writing challenges unique to these times.

Most of all we want to acknowledge our families (husbands Thomas and Pender), children (Diana, Thomas, John, Katherine, Linda, and Stan with spouses/partners Pedro, Chelsea, Szilvia, Patrick, Mikaela), and grandchildren (Natalia, Sophia, and Camryn) and step-grandchildren (Alex, Eric, and Victoria). While our husbands supported us throughout many late-night teaching sessions and even later writing sessions, it is for our children and grandchildren that the issues in this Framework are so critical. We care about their health now and in the future. Understanding the elements in the Framework may help to ensure a better health outcome for them and for all citizens in rural communities.

Chapter One

Overview of Rural Health Terms and Concepts

Introduction

The concepts pertaining to health and ideas regarding rural health are evident in published literature. Research and education sources are rich with discussions of what health is and is not. But perhaps only in the last 10 years is the concept of place as it relates to health the verity that living in a rural area impacts the health of rural populations. Rural health is becoming more frequently the topic of published literature. When reading about rural health we find it is often depicted through morbidity/mortality statistics, through gaps in services and resources, and through health disparities. This depiction of rural health does generate conversation about the health needs of rural areas, but it is dominated by what is lacking. As complex as rural health issues are, this deficit approach is insufficient to fully understand the nature of rural health and the elements that impact the health of people living in rural areas. A holistic and systematic approach to examining the health of people living in rural areas is essential to improved health outcomes (CDC, 2017).

In this chapter, we introduce the Rural Health Framework that provides the conceptual foundation upon which rural health issues are understood and upon which positive change can be realized by rural populations. In preparation for introducing the Rural Health Framework, we will explore eight terms and discuss the work of renowned researchers who helped advance our understanding of rural health. Beginning in this

Learning Outcomes

After reading Chapter 1, Overview of Rural Health Terms and Concepts, the learner will be able to

- Define the eight terms important to understanding Rural Health.
- Explain the rural health framework and the importance of the framework in improving the health of rural populations.

Key Topics

Learning about the following key topics will support you in achieving the chapter outcomes:

- **Rural Health Terms:** rural, health outcomes, health care access, interprofessional practice and education, health professional shortages, scopes of practice, licensure, certification.
- **Rural Health Concepts:** Holistic Theory and the Rural Health Framework.

first chapter and continuing in the chapters that follow, you will be immersed in a running case to pique your interest about the chapter content. Here is the running case for Chapter 1, Overview of Rural Health Terms and Concepts.

RUNNING CASE

Interprofessional Rural Health Training Program

In 1993, the federal government through a grant funding program that eventually would become the Quintin Burdick Interdisciplinary Rural Health Training program, funded university programs to teach health professions students interprofessional care. That year, a PharmD and an education specialist teamed to apply for such funding. Their project, the IRHE Rural Health Training Initiative, deviated from others awarded funding as it did not follow the more conventional path of developing university coursework to be delivered on campus. Instead, the project focused on bringing together students from multiple disciplines to live and learn together in a rural community. This immersion experience not only provided IPE learning for students, but also taught students about rural health. Equally important, the immersion project brought attention and resources to underserved rural communities.

Terms Important to Understanding Rural Health

In this chapter we want to familiarize you with terms that are critical to discussing and understanding **rural** health. Specifically, we will review what we mean by **rural**, **health outcome**, **health access**, **interprofessional practice and education**, **health professional shortages**, **scopes of practice** and, within that, the difference between **licensure and certification**. Following this review of terms, we will introduce the **Rural Health Framework** and the importance of the framework in improving the health of rural populations.

MEANING OF RURAL

As this book is about **rural** health, of course, the first thing we need to do is to define **"rural."** Easy? Well, not exactly. **Rural** can mean a lot of things to a lot of people. First, there are our own impressions of what we mean by **rural**.

Take a moment to describe for yourself what you picture when you hear the word **rural**. Over the years, we have asked students that same question. Their answers are remarkably similar. Some talk about the "rolling hills" or "farmland" or "wide-open spaces with lots of trees and few people." Many describe **rural** as "small towns" with "friendly people" "where everyone knows everyone else." Descriptions like this we often classify as density. In Chapter 2 we will delve more deeply into *density*, but for now we note that, for some, **rural** connotes low number of people.

Students also describe **rural** as a place one must leave in order to have more resources. These students say if you live in a **rural** area you have "to go into the big city" to "go to a large mall" or to "go to the movies" or to "go to a hospital." In this scenario, **rural** is something other than a larger city. For our purposes, we have grouped such descriptors as *proximity*, as in **rural** areas are in proximity to more resources found in larger cities. Our most succinct students simply say that "**rural** is not the big city," describing **rural** by *exclusion* of what it is not (a big city). While these students' descriptors are markedly similar, the descriptors also mirror official definitions. While there is not a single entity that defines **rural**, the definitions provided by three agencies are most often used as the standard definition of **rural**.

Secondly, there are official definitions of **rural**. For instance, the federal government defines rural. According to its publications, the **Census Bureau** starts by defining urban areas (areas with 50,000 or more people) and urban clusters (populations between 2,500 and less than 50,000). Everything that is not urban by these definitions is considered **rural** (U. S. Census Bureau, 2020). The **Office of Management and Budget** (OMB) uses a similar classification with designations of Metropolitan and Micropolitan areas similar to the Census Bureau's urban and urban cluster designations. That is, the Census Bureau and OMB classifies **rural** as anything not Metropolitan or Micropolitan (HRSA, 2020). More expansive than definitions provided by either the Census Bureau or OMB is that provided by the **Department of Agriculture, Economic Research Service**. Their definition includes elements of geography (e.g., open countryside) and population density (e.g. area with less than 2,500 people or with populations of less than 50,000 and not park of larger area) (USDA ERS, 2019). Their definition goes on to further refine **rural** through a series of codes (e.g., commuting areas or typology codes) (USDA ERS).

Thirdly, there are state agencies that define **rural**, researchers and research institutes that define **rural**, and the general public or elected leaders that define **rural**. Often, **rural** is defined by shared beliefs or practices, by general impressions and commonly held views, and by sociological factors that describe populations or settings in similar fashions.

As we see, there is no one uniformly agreed-upon definition of **rural**. This means that while many of us would say that we "know **rural** when we see it," we must constantly verify how a publication, agency, or program defines the term to ensure that we understand what is being communicated. For our purposes, we will define **rural** by using some elements of official definitions and some borrowed by the perceptions of people who intuitively define **rural** with components of economics, geographical, demographical and cultural elements. Thus, our definition of **rural** is an area with a population density of between 2,500 and less than 50,000 that has geographical/economic/cultural elements often associated with **rural**.

How rural is defined and who defines it is important. At the very least, it matters so that we can understand what others are saying. For instance, when a reporter says that people are migrating from urban areas to rural areas, we often have in mind people living in a large city like New York City migrating to an open-space, tranquil setting like Breckenridge, Colorado. But does the image also bring to mind New Yorkers moving to remote areas in Bayou County or isolated islands like Ocracoke? Probably not. We have in our minds what we mean, and without clarification of what the reporter has in mind, we are likely to incorrectly interpret news, reports, documents, or conversations.

When foundations and health care watch groups report that rural areas have difficulty attracting health care professionals, are they referring to attracting health care professionals to Palm Springs (population 44,552) or The Hamptons (population 58,261) where respectively the average house costs $415,300 and $1.1 million (City of Palm Springs, 2020), (Point2, n.d.), (Palm Springs, CA, n.d.), (CNBC)? More likely, the shortages are in less affluent, but similar-sized communities (around 50,000) where the average homes are a more modestly priced at $140,000.

Thus, knowing who is defining rural and how rural is defined matters. This became very clear during the pandemic. According to the Census Bureau, nearly 19 million people reside in rural areas. Media reports in early summer of 2020 demonstrated that rural areas were hit hard with disparate impact. But did these numbers include resort, luxury areas, and if so, was the impact even more intensified for less affluent, less well-connected, and lesser known rural areas? In our framework, we looked beyond population numbers, density, proximity, or even perceived ideas of rural as we utilized the factors and elements that make comparisons possible and meaningful.

> ## APPLICATION OPPORTUNITY
>
> Find two cities in your state that are similar in size but that have vastly different average housing costs or average incomes. Describe how these two would have different experiences recruiting health professionals to their area.

HEALTH OUTCOMES

A significant issue when discussing **rural** health is the fact that **rural** populations suffer worse **health outcomes** than urban populations. What do we mean when we use the term "**health outcomes**"? Many definitions are offered by various health care organizations and measurement services. Some definitions are expansive, as in improvement in patient's quality of life (Canadian Institute for Health Information) other definitions take a patient focus perspective, as in defining **health outcomes** to be the realization of patient expectations when seeking care—in other words what is most important to the patient (Institute for Strategy & Competitiveness). For our purposes we will combine definitions from the Center for Disease Control and Prevention and the World Health Organization and utilize the term *health outcomes to mean those measurements that include being alive; functioning well mentally, physically and socially and having* *a sense of well-being that are attributed to health interventions* (Parrish, 2010). We will revisit this issue several times throughout the book.

RUNNING CASE

Interprofessional Rural Health Training Program

By living in the community, students were able to experience nuances of rural culture and the meaning of relationships in a small town. This certainly was the case when, in the first rotation, a student went shopping for groceries at the locally owned store. Arriving at the checkout, the student realized she had left her checkbook at home (this was before the days of cards or phone apps). She apologized to the cashier about her forgetfulness as she gathered up her groceries to restock them.

"You're one of the health students living at the AHEC house, aren't you?" The cashier asked the student.

"Yes, we just arrived."

"Well, we are sure glad to have you all here," replied the cashier, "and don't worry about paying today. Just pay us the next time you're in. We sure are glad you all are here."

Relationships are everything in rural areas, or so the student learned on her first day of rotation.

HEALTH CARE ACCESS

Rural residents have worse **health outcomes** than their urban counterparts. One reason may be that **rural** residents lack access to health services, programs, and resources. Stop for a moment and ask yourself the question, why would **rural** residents have limited access to health services and health care? If you are like some of our students, you would say that they lack access because there is no hospital in the town or because the nearest specialist is so far away. And while that is true, lack of immediately available resources is one dimension of access; there are two other dimensions that contribute equally to preventing **rural** residents from having optimum opportunity for healthier outcomes.

One agency that has advocated for greater **health access** is the World Health Organization (WHO). According to the WHO, access has three dimensions: physical accessibility, financial affordability, and acceptability (Evans, 2013). The WHO definition is consistent with that of the US Healthy People.gov, which defines **health access** as having entry into the health system through insurance and other financial considerations, geographical availability of services, and a personal relationship with providers that is based on trust and communication

According to the World Health Organization (WHO) health access includes. ...

- Physical accessibility. This is understood as the availability of good health services within reasonable reach of those who need them, along with opening hours, appointment systems, and other aspects of service organization and delivery that allow people to obtain services when they need them.

- Financial affordability. This is a measure of people's ability to pay for services without financial hardship. It takes into account not only the price of the health services but also indirect costs and opportunity costs (e.g., the costs of transportation to and from facilities and of taking time away from work). Affordability is influenced by the wider health financing system and by household income.

- Acceptability. This captures people's willingness to seek services. Acceptability is low when patients perceive services to be ineffective or when social and cultural factors such as language or the age, sex, ethnicity, or religion of the health provider discourage them from seeking services (Evans, 2013).

(Office of Disease Prevention and Health Promotion, 2020). Thus, **health access** can be denied because of lack of services or because patients do not have the means to afford the services when they are available. Equally important, access does not exist when people do not have financial means to use these services (they have no insurance, cannot afford to take time off work, cannot afford treatments), and when there is no trust with providers or patients cannot communicate with providers.

INTERPROFESSIONAL EDUCATION AND PRACTICE (IPE)

Proponents of IPE emerged as early as 1969. Touted as a means of utilizing limited resources, IPE received considerable traction in 1988 with the U. S. Government backing The Health Professions Reauthorization Act, which became known as the Quentin N. Burdick Rural Health Interdisciplinary Grant Program. While the focus of this grant program was to bring IPE to **rural** areas, the IPE was from its inception a global movement, with very strong advocates in the UK and Canada. Today, organizations like the Center for the Advancement of Interprofessional Education (CAIPE) based in the U.K. and the National Center for Interprofessional Practice and Education in the US serve as think tanks, repositories of curriculum and research, and conveners to help educate future health professionals in interprofessional and collaborative education and care. The National Center for Interprofessional Practice and Education also supports the incorporation of IPE Core Competencies, first developed in 2009 and updated in 2016, into educational accreditation standards of most health professions (IEC, 2016).

RUNNING CASE

Interprofessional Rural Health Training Program

An important part of caring for rural patients is knowing the patient: who they are, where they live, their support system, the resources they have and don't have. To help students understand their patients, two students each week visited a patient in the patient's home. Often these visits extended to meeting family members and even neighbors. Patients were delighted to tell their stories, and students began to understand that the burden of disease often extends far beyond the person diagnosed with the illness. Students learned the importance of walking an extra mile in a rural setting.

In **rural** areas, IPE makes sense. Working collaboratively with other professionals maximizes scarce resources, reduces professional isolation (often a contributing factor to professional burnout), and contributes to enhanced quality of care. Valuable knowledge and skill are utilized when the patient's physician, nurses, pharmacist, and social worker at the **rural** hospital collaborate regarding the plan of care during bedside rounds. Professionals from different health disciplines share their prospective in regard to the patient's well-being. They are educationally prepared to consider the whole patient. Their discussion includes the patient's biophysical needs as well as social, cultural, and spiritual needs. The patient and family are part of planning for the desired health outcome. Further consultation can occur, perhaps through telehealth, to provide a higher level of care for a patient than is available at the **rural** hospital.

> The term **interdisciplinary** was originally used until the CAIPE definition of **Interprofessional Education**. Today, the term IPE stands for **Interprofessional Practice and Education** to encompass how health-related professionals learn and work (NCIPE, n.d.).
>
> IPE: The accepted definition of IPE occurs when "professions to learn from, with and about one another ... with the [objective] of cultivating collaborative practice" (Barr, 2018).

Interprofessional

We mention one caution: interprofessional care is sometimes referred to as interprofessional team-based care. We have avoided that term for a variety of reasons. First, students often think of teams in terms of sports illustration. For instance, students think of a team as a basketball team—a tightly knit group of individuals who work seamlessly to master the goal of winning. Students see such a team as unified and fluid in its movements and, most importantly, as working as a single unit, together in the same place at the same time. These types of teams certainly exist in health care. For instance, there are tightly coordinated teams working in a Rehabilitation or a Behavioral Medicine Units. But there are other kinds of teams—a football team composed of various squads that come together when needed or a gymnastics team composed of individual competitors. You can also substitute an orchestra or band for a sports analogy. The issue is that our first impression of what constitutes a "team" might prevent us from looking at the variety of teams that exist around us.

Second, we have avoided using the term "team" in conjunction with interprofessional because students have a tendency to think of a team as bound by place and time. Teams gather in a specific place (e.g., conference room, a field) at a given time. But that is not always the case—think of virtual teams that span across the globe. In rural areas, interprofessional care teams may be unbounded by the time and space concept.

Let's imagine for a moment a rural community with a pharmacist in a retail store, a provider in a clinic, and a social worker in the community health department. Let's further imagine that patients have electronic health records that allow quick and easy communication among providers in an area. So, on a given day, the pharmacist notices that a patient who regularly has prescriptions refilled has been missing refills. The pharmacist alerts the clinic of this. The provider reviews the message and asks the case manager in the clinic to follow up with the patient. In doing so, the case manager learns that the patient who is on a fixed income has had some expected expenses recently: a major roof repair and car repairs. To save money, the patient has been splitting the pills so they will last longer. The case manager contacts the social worker, who works with the patient to find medication grants to offset prescription costs. In this scenario, the constellation of professionals worked collaboratively, communicating through existing media without coming together in time and place. This may be the more realistic model for interprofessional work in underserved rural areas.

Primary care includes physicians in family medicine, pediatrics, general internal medicine, obstetrics–gynecology; mental health includes physicians in psychiatry and all core mental health providers (clinical social psychologists, clinical social workers, psychiatric nurse specialists, marriage and family therapists); dental includes general dentists and dental auxiliaries (Health Resources & Services Administration, May 2020).

HEALTH PROFESSIONAL SHORTAGES

Because of limited access issues for **rural** residents, **rural** communities must maximize resources. This is certainly true in health care where there are both **health professional shortages** and a need to leverage those resources as much as possible. Most underserved areas lack enough health professionals to serve their populations at the desired care level. Chronic shortages include physicians, dentists, nurses, pharmacists, nutritionists, and diabetic educators, just to name a few. While insufficient numbers of all health professionals are important, the federal government has identified those areas that lack primary care, mental health, and general dental professions. Using scoring criteria such as provider–population ratio, poverty level percentages, and travel time to nearest source of care, the Health Resources and Service Administration, a

> **APPLICATION OPPORTUNITY**
>
> Review the designation Medically Underserved Area and Medically Underserved Population (MUA/P). Go to: https://bhw.hrsa.gov/shortage-designation/hpsa-criteria
> Compare the distinction of MUA/P to HPSA designations.

federal agency, calculates a score qualifying an area to be designated a Health Professional Shortage Area (HPSA) (Health Resources & Services Administration, May 2020). Designation of a HPSA makes the area/facility/population eligible to receive some designated funding, assistance in recruiting and retaining professionals, or Medicare bonus payments.

SCOPE OF PRACTICE

One important aspect of working collaboratively in an interprofessional team setting is understanding what others on the team do. This knowledge is particularly significant in **rural** areas that may have professional shortages and that seek to maximize the expertise of available professionals. We sometimes refer to this understanding of others as a professional's "scope of practice." For our purposes, we will say that **scope of practice** includes those tasks that a professional can perform and has authority to perform. In order to understand the "can perform" and "authority to perform" we have to review two concepts: **licensure and certification**.

At its most basic distinction, **licensure** is the permission that an agency of the government grants a person to perform a specified set of skills. For instance, a state licenses a nurse to perform specified tasks, such as conducting a nursing assessment within its jurisdiction. Likewise, a state licenses a physician, a pharmacist, or a physical therapist, to name a few licensed professions. The state may delegate the actual review and determination of compliance with licensing requirements to a board (as in the case of having the Board of Nursing review licensing requirements for RNs and LPNs). But regardless of who reviews, the state is awarding a license as permission to practice in that state.

> **Licensure** is the state's grant of legal authority to practice a profession within a designated scope of practice (National Registry of Emergency Medical Technicians).

> **Certification** is an attestation of the skills that a professional has gained to perform a set of tasks.

Certification, on the other hand, speaks to the skills or competency that an individual must have to complete a set of tasks. **Certification** can be granted by an educational institution or a professional association. Examples of **certification** include a physician obtaining a Board Certification in Pediatrics through the American College of Pediatrics or a nurse receiving Nursing Certification in Critical Care through the American Association of Critical Care Nursing. In both examples the professional was licensed and then received the **certification** as attestation to the special skills that they had (skills in pediatrics; skills in critical care nursing) (Department of Health, Education, and Welfare, 1971).

APPLICATION OPPORTUNITY

Pick a profession. Explore the requirements (education program/degree, license, certification) needed for that profession. Describe the tasks that the professional may perform. Also explore where the professional may practice. Share your findings with classmates.

Returning to the concept of **Scope of Practice**, then, we mean by **Scope of Practice** the set of skills that a professional may perform within their area of expertise, as defined by **licensure** and/or **certification**. **Scopes of practice**, especially when accompanied by **licensure** requirements, are written in a legal practice act. This act spells out both the skills that the professional can perform and the requirements to maintain **licensure** (e.g., continuing education requirements, legal constraints, etc.). It is critically important in **rural**, underserved areas that professionals "practice at the top of their scope of practice"—that is that professionals are working at the maximum of their capabilities. To do less is to waste a valuable and limited resource.

Section Review

In this section we discussed eight terms that help us to understand Rural Health. We considered our own personal definitions of **rural** and then compared it to that of three official entities that define **rural**. Next, we explored the terms **health access** and **health outcomes** as they pertain to **rural** health. The terms **IPE** and **health professional shortages** we defined and discussed in relationship to health resources for **rural** areas. Furthering the discussion of meeting health resource needs, we explored **scope of practice** and contrasted **licensure** with **certification**.

RUNNING CASE

Interprofessional Rural Health Training Program

The IRHE Rural Health Training Initiative depended on the assistance of a committed on-campus advisory board and the help of loyal community partners (including a community health center, Eastern Area Health Center, and local preceptors). The design was to bring together students who were already enrolled in a discipline-specific rotation in rural communities for one day of intensive rural health interprofessional education. Ultimately, over the program's 12-year history, three rural hubs were established, a dozen professions from multiple universities participated in the program, three AHEC houses accommodated the students, hundreds of rural patients were seen, and thousands of rural immersion hours were clocked. Lots of learning occurred, not the least of which was learning relative to the health issues and concerns faced by rural populations.

LEARNING ASSESSMENT—RURAL HEALTH TERMS

Take this Learning Assessment, and then compare your responses to the answers provided at the end of the book. You may find there are terms pertaining to rural health that you would like to review to gain a better understanding.

1. Rural health issues are simplistic and do not require a holistic and systematic approach in order to achieve improved health outcomes in rural populations. (True/False)
2. List three organizations that provide an official definition of "rural."
3. The WHO tells us that health care access is three-dimensional. List these three dimensions of health care access.
4. Once a nurse graduates from an accredited nursing school, what other credential must that nurse obtain before practicing?
5. Provide an example of an organization that offers certifications to nurses.

Theoretical and Conceptual Constructs and Frameworks to Date

When looking toward a conceptual framework for rural health, we must turn our attention to holistic thinking and to Australia. Holistic thinking provides the conceptual premise upon which the Rural Health Framework is based. Two Australian researchers, Lisa Bourke and Jane Farmer, are well published as advocates for creating theoretical frameworks to address rural and remote health. The Rural Health Framework draws upon their published work.

HOLISTIC THINKING

Borrowing concepts from systems thinking, holistic thinking requires that issues be viewed as interrelated and interlocking elements that influence and are influenced by other elements. That is, instead of concentrating on analyzing part of a system (e.g., lack of **health access** caused by shortages of health personnel), we must incorporate all the sub-elements that impact the issue (e.g., lack of **health access** caused by shortages, distrust, unfair burden of care, geographical placement of personnel). At its most basic level, holistic thinking is being able to see the whole complex system while understanding the interdependent parts (Lebcir, 2006). Our Rural Health Framework depicts a holistic approach to understanding the interrelatedness of the factors and elements that influence outcomes, access to health care, and health status in rural areas.

THEORIES AND FRAMEWORKS

Although at times the terms are used interchangeably, "theory" and "framework" are two distinct concepts. This section begins with a definition of "theory" and explores the need for and proposed theories relative to rural health, including theories from other disciplines that might be useful in formulating a rural health theory. The second part of this section explores the meaning of "framework" and gives examples of how frameworks have been developed to plan and allocate resources relative to rural health. This section provides background information that informs a discussion of the Rural Health Framework, which is the basis for this book.

Theory

Many sophisticated definitions of "theory" exist. For instance, Kerlinger and Lee define theory as "a set of interrelated constructs (concepts), definitions, and propositions that present a systematic view of phenomena by specifying relations among variables, with the purpose of explaining and predicting the phenomena" (Kerlinger and Lee, 2000). More simply, the *American Heritage Dictionary* defines theory as "a set of statements or principles devised to explain a group of facts or phenomena, especially one that has been repeatedly tested or is widely accepted and can be used to make predictions about natural phenomena."

Thus, we see that theory requires (a) statements or principles or constructs that (b) explain and predict phenomena and that have (c) been tested or utilized sufficiently to make the understanding and prediction accepted by others. Theory development explains, fosters understanding, helps predict phenomena, and serves to verify that phenomena. What about a rural health theory? Is there a widely accepted theory that defines and predicts the phenomena of rural health?

Rural Health Theory

As with most academic research, we start by conducting a review of literature to see what has been published on rural health theory. When we did such a search, we found a couple of interesting facts: 1) there does not seem to be an accepted rural health theory; and 2) Australian researchers have led the way in espousing a need for rural health theory and in proposing conceptual tenets for inclusion.

In 2010, well-known and respected Australian rural health researchers argued the need for theory development specific to rural and remote health. Noting lack of academic programs devoted to rural health or a defined field of study or discipline in rural health, the researchers nevertheless argued forcefully for greater attention to rural health theory development. For one, theory would guide how future practitioners and researchers studied rural health and the corresponding health issues. For another, theory would enable a degree of predictability stemming from comprehensive understanding of rural health articulated through key assumptions germane to the topic (Bourke et al., 2010b).

In addition to championing the need for theory development, Australian researchers identified key concepts that could eventually be incorporated into a rural health theory. Those discussed included community, social capital, and social determinants of health. For some, a relational model seemed appropriate for examining and understanding rural health. As was stated "what typifies public perceptions of 'rural health' is *poorer health status*, especially among indigenous Australians, *poorer access to healthcare* and the *lack of staff*, particularly doctors" (Bourke et al., 2010a). Other consistent themes emerging from rural health research were the tendency for *relationship-based service provision* (Farmer, 2007), where clients and providers know each other (and may overlap), and the role of health services in *community sustainability* (Farmer et al., 2003).

Another model, based upon Gidden's theory of structuration and the interplay of structure and agency, incorporated into its model the health concepts of 1) geographic isolation, 2) the rural locale, 3) local health responses, 4) broader health systems, 5) social structures, and 6) power (Bourke et al.,2012). Other researchers added community sustainability. Still others sought to develop a theory that would recognize the intersection of people, politics, environment, history, and economic opportunity (Farmer et al., 2012).

Certainly, the complexity of a health care system with its multidisciplinary nature and interrelated variables dictates a holistic approach to analysis, resource allocation, and improved outcomes. Coupled with the need for a more robust and comprehensive view of rural, the need for new rural health theory becomes apparent. While no single rural health theory is currently endorsed by researchers, the journey for theory development continues. The reason, as Farmer (2012) so eloquently stated, is that "a rural health theory might lead us to understand rural health as a set of issues, to innovate with methodology and to explore new avenues" (Farmer et al., 2012). Perhaps looking at other disciplines for theory assistance might help.

Borrowing From Other Disciplines

Espoused theories within specific disciplines guide practitioners and researchers and offer a potential candidate for understanding rural health issues and outcomes. For instance, the ecological model found in health behavior and disease prevention literature seeks to integrate various components (individual, population, community) through a series of relationships that acknowledges the interaction of these relationships upon health, health behavior, and health outcome (Ecological Models of Health Behavior and Health Promotion, n.d.). Likewise, the Health Belief Model again found in National Center for Health Promotion and Disease Prevention literature seeks to predict individual health behavior by focusing on individual beliefs such as perceived susceptibility, perceived severity of an illness, as well as perceived benefits and barriers to action (Rural Health Information Hub). Both theories could help to inform behaviors and domains critical to understanding rural health issues and outcomes.

Particularly robust have been rural health theories developed within the nursing discipline. As early as 1989, Long and Weinert (1989), concerned about the unique issues and needs of rural populations, identified key concepts pertinent to rural populations: work beliefs, isolation and distance, and self-reliance In 2018, Winters and Lee published their first edition of *Rural Nursing: Concepts, Theory, and Practice* in which they expanded on the issues outlined in 1989. In their chapter on the development of theory, the authors describe the interdisciplinary nature of collaboration among researchers in the development of middle range theory to guide rural health nursing practice. Key to the theory was the demand that practitioners understand the unique issues and concerns facing rural populations (Winters & Lee, 2018).

Framework

Leaving theory, let's turn our attention to framework. Again, we turn to the *American Heritage Dictionary* that provides a general definition of framework: A set of assumptions, concepts, values, and practices that constitutes a way of viewing reality. We also like the *Cambridge Dictionary* definition that extends the meaning of framework to include a particular set of rules, ideas, or beliefs which you use in order to deal with problems or to decide what to do (*Collins English Dictionary*, n.d.). By these two definitions we see that frameworks are a way of (a) arraying concepts to (b) view a phenomenon sometimes for the purpose of (c) dealing with problems or (d) deciding on action. Certainly, we can see evidence of how rural health frameworks have been used to plan and plan interventions.

The Australian Government Department of Health in 2011 published the Australian Rural Health Strategic Planning Framework as a blueprint for action in improving health in rural and remote areas. Five principle domains were identified: access, service model and models of care, health workforce, collaborative partnerships and planning, and strong leadership, governance, transparency and performance. Under each domain action plans, resources, implications/requirements, and/or outcomes measures were articulated and described. For instance, under the domain of health workforce three goals were established, including improved availability of training and continuing professional development programs for rural and remote health professionals. Five action plans were described, including targeting training placement sites in areas of great workforce needs and development of funding mechanisms for distance supervision (page 36, Department of Health | National Strategic Framework for Rural and Remote Health). Working through the framework, the Australian government hoped to establish a coordinated and effective service delivery for its rural and remote areas.

In 2020, the U.S. Department of Health and Human Services published its "Four-Point Strategy to Transform Rural Health and Human Services." Aimed at addressing the challenges faced by rural communities while highlighting potential opportunities to improve rural health and human service outcomes, the framework identified four areas of emphasis, including: 1) Build a Sustainable Health and Human Services Model for Rural Communities by empowering rural providers to transform service delivery on a broad scale. 2) Leverage Technology and Innovation to deliver quality care and services to rural communities more efficiently and cost-effectively. 3) Focus on Preventing Disease and Mortality by developing rural-specific efforts to improve health outcomes. 4) Increase Rural Access to Care by eliminating regulatory burdens that limit the availability of needed clinical professionals (Australian Government Department of Health (2011) Australian Rural Health Strategic Planning Framework, p. 14). The intent of this planning framework was to ensure coordinated efforts across the Department of Health and Human Services through greater awareness of health and human services issues faced by rural populations, identification of gaps that the Department could address collaboratively, and development of policy or programs that would demonstrate how HHS was addressing rural challenges. Like the Australian Strategic Planning Framework, the U.S. Four-Point Strategy Framework served as a comprehensive planning tool (Rural Action Plan, 2020).

APPLICATION OPPORTUNITY

Explore the literature for other rural health theories and/or frameworks. Describe the foundational premise upon which the theory/framework is based and the major tenets of the theory/framework.

THE RURAL HEALTH FRAMEWORK

This holistic framework is based on our belief that the health status and health care access of people living in rural areas can best be examined and the most appropriate interventions implemented when five factors and 25 elements are analyzed specific to the rural area under consideration. The five factors are the geographical factor, the economical factor, the demographical factor, the sociocultural factor, and the support factor. The five factors are often depicted graphically.

For simplicity of presentation, factors form the first tier of the framework—the thematic divisions. Under each factor are five elements that define and delineate what is meant by the factor. It is at the element level that data is collected and comparisons are made. The elements provide a systematic and holistic analysis of topics that impact rural health. Depicted graphically, the factors and elements look like this:

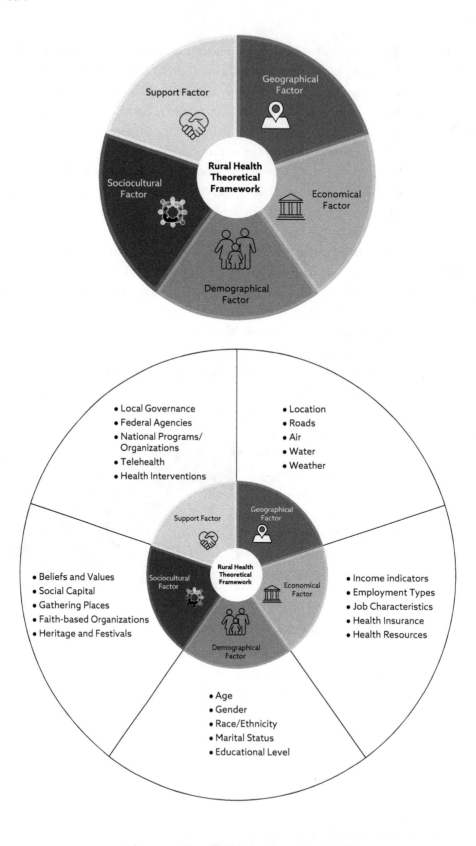

While this presentation helps us learn about the five factors and 25 elements, in reality, the interaction between factors and elements is much more complex. Elements within a factor interact with one another to intensify effects (e.g., poor roads and weather) while elements across factors deepen understanding of and appreciate the intertwining effect of issues (e.g., shortage of providers with changing demographics). In the coming chapters, we shall study each factor and element separately. However, as we proceed in the book, we shall begin to draw together elements to demonstrate the interaction that occurs and must be accounted for in order to understand the complexity that is rural health.

Section Review

In this section we examined concepts and theories that have advanced our insight into rural health issues. We learned that the Rural Health Framework depicts a holistic approach of examining the complexity and interconnectedness of factors that influence health outcomes as well as health care access in rural areas.

RUNNING CASE

Interprofessional Rural Health Training Program

Students, however, could not learn rural culture, economics, demographics, or environment without the assistance of an on-site teacher. Key to the student's learning was a faculty member who lived in the community and who became their learning guide, cultural translator, and rural health professor. Over the course of the 12 years that the IRHT program was operational, the rural health students saw and connected with the issues critical to understanding rural health. They learned from faculty members who served as community preceptors, teaching students, inviting them into their homes, asking students to accompany them on community outings, and even looking in on students as they experienced their first hurricanes.

The faculty's detailed notes of observations, reflections, feedback, and lessons learned enabled them to translate lessons learned in the community into undergraduate and graduate coursework taught on campus. Since the first course offering, rural health has been taught to thousands of students. Each class further refined and affirmed the insights gained about rural health. From this collective experience, the Rural Health Framework was developed to capture the breadth of issues necessary to impact health in rural settings. This framework is presented in the chapters that follow.

LEARNING ASSESSMENT—RURAL HEALTH CONCEPTS

Take this Learning Assessment, and then compare your responses to the answers provided at the end of the book. You may find there are rural health concepts you would like to review to gain a better understanding.

1. Holistic thinking is being able to see the whole system, while understanding the interdependent parts.
   a. True
   b. False
2. Name the two Australian rural health researchers who advocate for theory development to understand rural and remote health better.
3. How many factors and how many elements comprise the Rural Health Framework?
4. List the five factors that comprise the Rural Health Framework.
5. At what level in the Rural Health Framework is data collected?

CHAPTER SUMMARY

In this first chapter, we present an overview of terms to facilitate our exploration of rural health. Through defining seven terms and applying them to rural health we have begun to outline the complex nature of health concerns facing rural populations. In fact, we acknowledge the complexity in defining "rural" itself. Briefly, we lay out the Rural Health Framework along with foundational scholarly works leading to the development of this framework. The following chapters are organized based upon this framework. It is our hope that you will find this framework a logical and holistic process for understanding the complexity of health issues and concerns of rural populations.

REFERENCES—TERMS

Barr, H. (2018, March 25). Interprofessional education: What, how & when? CAIPE Bulletin Nos. 13 (1997) https://www.caipe.org/resources/publications/archived-publications/caipe-bulletin-nos-13-1997-interprofessional-education-what-how-when

Canadian Institute for Health Information. (n.d.). Outcomes. https://www.cihi.ca/en/outcomes

Centers for Disease Control and Prevention. (2017, August 2). About rural health. https://www.cdc.gov/ruralhealth/about.html

CNBC. (July 23,2020). Home prices in the Hamptons hit record as wealthy New Yorkers flee to the beach.https://www.cnbc.com/2020/07/23/coronavirus-home-prices-in-hamptons-hit-record-as-wealthy-new-yorkers-flee.html

City of Palm Springs, California. (January 16, 2020). Housing profile. [pdf]. https://www
.palmspringsca.gov/home/showdocument?id=71742

Evans, D. B., Hsu, J. & Boerma, T. (2013). Universal health coverage and universal access. *Bulletin of the World Health Organization, 91,* 546–546A. https://www.who.int/bulletin/ volumes/91/8/13-125450/en/

Health Resources & Services Administration. (2020, May). Shortage designation application and review process. https://bhw.hrsa.gov/shortage-designation/application-review-process

Health Resources & Services Administration. (2020, May). Shortage designation scoring criteria. https://bhw.hrsa.gov/shortage-designation/hpsa-criteria

Health Resources & Services Administration. (2020, July). Defining rural population. https:// www.hrsa.gov/rural-health/about-us/definition/index.html

Institute for Strategy & Competitiveness. (n.d.) International consortium for health outcomes measurement. https://www.isc.hbs.edu/about-michael-porter/affiliated-organizations-in- stitutions/pages/ichom.aspx

Interprofessional Education Collaborative. (2016). *Core competencies for interprofessional collaborative practice: 2016 update.* Interprofessional Education Collaborative. [pdf]. https:// hsc.unm.edu/ipe/resources/ipec-2016-core-competencies.pdf

Kerlinger, F. N., & Lee, H. B. (2000). *Foundations of behavioural research.* 4th ed. Cengage Learning.

National Center for Interprofessional Practice and Education. (n.d.). About interprofessional practice and education. https://nexusipe.org/informing/about-ipe

National Registry of Emergency Medical Technicians. (n.d.). Legal differences between certifi- cation and licensure. https://www.nremt.org/rwd/public/document/certification_licensure

Office of Disease Prevention and Health Promotion. (2020, August 18). Access to health services. https://www.healthypeople.gov/2020/topics-objectives/topic/Access-to-Health -Services

Palm Springs, California. (n.d.). Cost of living in Palm, Springs, California. https://www .bestplaces.net/cost_of_living/city/california/palm_springs

Parrish, R. G. (2010). Measuring population health outcomes. *Preventing Chronic Disease, 7*(4), A71. https://www.cdc.gov/Pcd/issues/2010/jul/10_0005.htm

Point2. (n.d.). The Hamptons –South Fork demographics. https://www.point2homes.com/US/ Neighborhood/NY/The-Hamptons-South-Fork-Demographics.html

United States Census Bureau. (2020, February 24). Urban and rural. https://www.census.gov/ programs-surveys/geography/guidance/geo-areas/urban-rural.html

United States Department of Agriculture Economic Research Service. (2019, October 23). Overview. https://www.ers.usda.gov/topics/rural-economy-population/rural-classifications/

United States Department of Agriculture Economic Research Service. (2019, October 23). https://www.ers.usda.gov/data-products/county-typology-codes/

United States Department of Health, Education, and Welfare (1971, June). Report on licensure and related health personnel credentialing. https://eric.ed.gov/?id=ED061420

Well-Ahead. (n.d.). Health professional shortage areas. https://www.walpen.org/hpsa

REFERENCES—CONCEPTS

Australian Government Department of Health. (2011). Australian rural health strategic planning framework [pdf]. https://www1.health.gov.au/internet/main/publishing.nsf/Content/national-strategic-framework-rural-remote-health#:~:text=The%20National%20Strategic%20Framework%20for%20Rural%20and%20Remote%20Health%20promotes,in%20rural%20and%20remote%20communities.&text=Overall%20it%20aims%20to%20improve,for%20rural%20and%20remote%20Australians

Bourke, L., Coffin, J., Taylor, J., & Fuller, J. (2010a). Rural health in Australia. *Rural Society: The Journal of Research Into Rural and Regional Social Issues in Australia, 20*(1), 2–9.

Bourke, L., Humphreys, J. S., Wakerman, J., & Taylor, J. (2010b, March 24). Charting the future course of rural health and remote health in Australia: Why we need theory. *Australian Journal of Rural Health, 18*(2), 54–58.

Bourke, L., Humphreys, J. S., Wakeman, J., & Taylor, J. (2012). Understandong rural and remote health: A framework for analysis in Australia. *Health & Place, 18*(3), 496–503.

Collins English Dictionary. (n.d.). Framework. https://www.collinsdictionary.com/us/dictionary/english/conceptual-framework

Ecological Models of Health Behavior and Health Promotion (n.d.). PDF, EPUB. am-medicine.com)

Farmer J. (2007). Connected care in a fragmented world: Lessons from rural health care. *The British Journal of General Practice : The Journal of the Royal College of General Practitioners, 57*(536), 225–230.

Farmer, J., Lauder, W., Richards, H., & Sharkey, S. (2003). Dr. John has gone: Assessing health professionals' contribution to remote rural community sustainability in the UK. *Social Science & Medicine, 57*(4), 673– 686.

Farmer, J., Munoz, S. A., & Threlkeld, G. (2012). Theory in rural health. *The Australian Journal of Rural Health, 20*, 185–189.

Lebcir, R. (2006). Health care management: The contribution of systems thinking. https://uhra.herts.ac.uk/bitstream/handle/2299/683/S65.pdf

Long, K. A., & Weinert C. (1989, Summer). Rural nursing: Developing the theory base. *Sch Inq Nurs Pract, 3*(2), 113–27.

Rural Health Information Hub. (n.d.). The health belief model. https://www.ruralhealthinfo.org/toolkits/health-promotion/2/theories-and-models/health-belief

U.S. Department of Health and Human Services. (2020). Rural action plan [pdf]. https://www
    .hhs.gov/sites/default/files/hhs-rural-action-plan.pdf
Winters, Charlene A., & Lee, Helen (eds.). (2018, March 13). *Rural nursing: Concepts, theory, and
    practice* (5th ed.). Springer Publishing Company.

Figure Credits

Chapter Two

The Geographical Factor

Introduction

The Rural Health Framework is structured around five factors that impact rural health. The five factors are the geographical factor, the economical factor, the demographical factor, the sociocultural factor, and the support factor, with the end result that the Rural Health Framework establishes a holistically systematic way to assess rural health care access and rural health status. When applying this framework in the assessment of rural health, the end result is an examination considering all the unique needs of an area and the people who live there.

In this chapter, we will explore the geographical factor. To thoroughly assess how the geographical factor influences the health of people living in rural areas, it is important to examine separately each of the elements comprising the geographical factor. Following this systematic method avoids the tendency to stray from the elements comprising the geographical factor and prematurely delve into issues unrelated to the geography of the rural area being assessed. Thus, we will be discussing the elements that comprise the geographical factor: location, roads, air, water, and weather and the health outcomes associated with each element. While we will discuss each element separately, we shall see how they integrate and multiply the effects of each other to form more complex issues that affect health outcomes, especially in rural areas. To humanize these issues, in this chapter we shall meet the Wheeler family and the impact that each element has on the family. At the end of the chapter, we

Learning Outcomes

After reading about the geographical factor, the learner will be able to

- Identify the five elements that comprise the geographical factor.
- Explain how each of the elements impacts the health status and/or health care access of people living in rural areas.
- Analyze and apply the geographical factor and the elements comprising the geographical factor in an assessment of their contribution to rural health outcomes.

Key Topics

Learning about the following key topics will support you in achieving the chapter outcomes:

- **Location:**
  topography, county seat, population density, and population centers
- **Roads:**
  design of rural roads, road shoulders, obstacles, vehicular accidents, and EMS response
- **Air:**
  unobstructed airflow and sources of air pollution
- **Water:**
  drinking water, runoff, vector-borne diseases, and recreational
- **Weather:**
  precipitation changes, flooding, heat-related illnesses, and cold-related illnesses

will explore how we can systematically collect geographical factor data through completion of an assessment grid that captures each of the elements and forms a comprehensive description of the geographical elements in a county or region.

RUNNING CASE

Wheeler Family

The Wheelers live on a farm down Highway 11. The family consists of Fred (age 43), Alice (age 41), and their two children, Sam (age 17) and Evie (age 14). Fred farms on land that has been in his family for three generations. Alice is a social worker at the County Health Department, located in Pineville about 45 minutes away. Both of their children attend the public high school, which is about 30 minutes from the Wheeler farm.

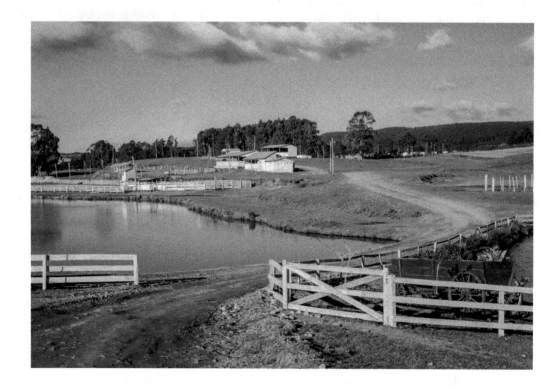

Location as an Element of the Geographical Factor

We don't have to think very hard to realize that location (of people and health care resources) matters. For one, we can look at a popular diagram showing the life expectancy of persons living along some geographical terrain. In our illustration we will use Highway 64 in eastern North Carolina, running from Wake County to Martin County as it passes through Franklin County, Nash County, and Edgecombe County. The life expectancy varies by seven years depending on whether one lives in Wake County or Martin County (Center on Society and Health, Virginia Commonwealth University, 2015).

We see from this simple example that a location along this highway may have significant implications and outcomes. While there are many variables that explain the difference in life expectancy along this corridor, the map shows that location is an important element in our thinking about health care outcomes. Let's dig deeper into this discussion of location.

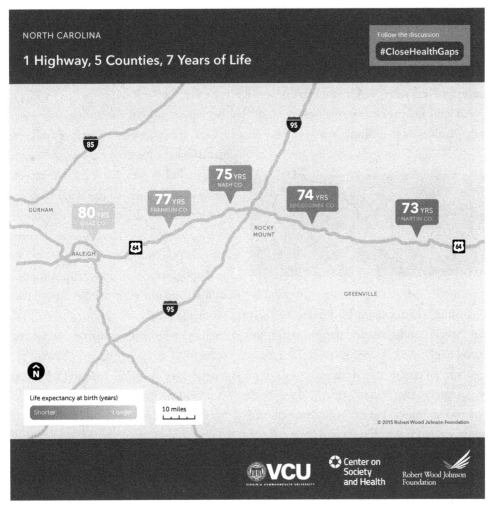

FIGURE 2.1   One Highway, Five Counties, Seven Years of Life.

When we talk about a geographical unit that we can use to compare one area to another, we find that much like "rural" there is not unified agreement on that geographical unit. Some researchers and planners rely on states as a geographical point of comparison. You can see that in data reported. Other researchers use zip codes as a geographical point, relying heavily on U.S. Census Bureau data. For our purposes, we will define the geographical unit of location element according to more governmental lines: counties, the geographical units used in 48 states, parishes used in Louisiana; and boroughs used in Alaska. For our purpose, we standardized the term to "county." Once we have the unit of geographical measure, we need to determine key components within that physical element. We will discuss how within the location element there are four key components: description of the topography of the county, county seat, population density within the county, and towns/population centers.

Topography is the layout of the physical features of a land area. Maps are used to represent topography. One can best examine the **topography** of an area by on-site surveying of the land.

Our first component in this element is **topography**. We know that topography means the physical features of a land area (*Cambridge Dictionary*, n.d.). Some areas are relatively flat, some hilly, some dry, and some wet. All land features work together to describe the topography of the area. Using eastern North Carolina as an example, we would say that eastern North Carolina is part of the coastal plains, with a variety of topographical features including low-lying areas at or below sea level, proximity to the Atlantic Ocean, presence of sounds, inner coastal waterways, rivers, swamps, wetlands, streams, forests, and open farmland.

APPLICATION OPPORTUNITY

Describe the topographical features of your county or region.

Topography is an important component of our location element because, among other things, the topography determines travel distance, travel time, and travel difficulty under typical conditions and in unusual situations such as inclement conditions. People need to travel to get to work or to go to health care appointments. Emergency services have to reach patients in an emergency. Those who live in areas where travel requires crossing a ferry that may not operate 24/7 or crossing bridges that may not be open during high wind conditions have a topographical barrier to accessing health services. Counties with land features such as swamps, wetlands, and forests will have vast areas that are void of development, leaving people who live in surrounding areas further distances to travel. Thus, knowledge of the **topography** is important.

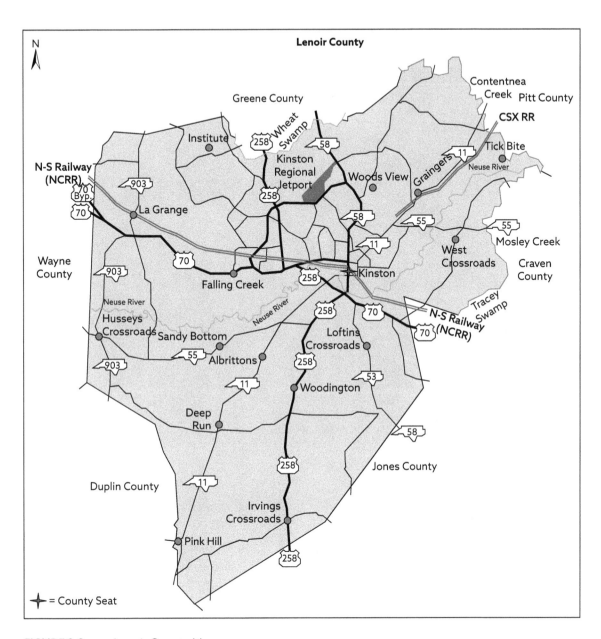

FIGURE 2.2a   Lenoir County Map.

Critical to understanding the relationship of health and location is the placement and access to resources. The **county seat** is the town that serves as the governmental center for the county.

The **county seat** is that town within the county that is the administrative and governmental center for the county.

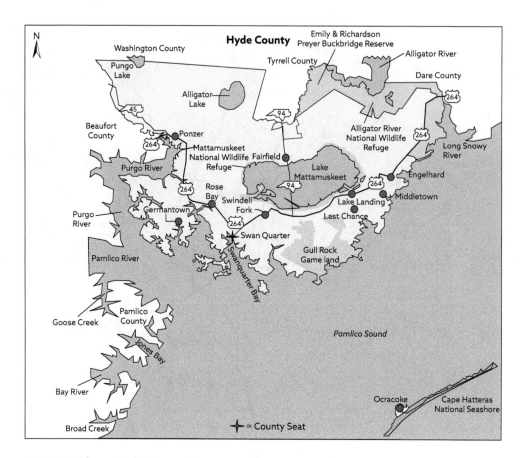

FIGURE 2.2b   Hyde County Map.

Often, health care and social services are concentrated in the **county seat**. Services found in the **county seat** are the hospital, health department, EMS, fire/rescue, sheriff's office, courthouse, social services, main post office, and the USDA Farm Service Agency. As important as the services found in the county are, the location of the **county seat** is also critically important to the citizens of the county (Ricketts, 2002).

The location of the **county seat** of a given county impacts the health care access of people living throughout the county. Ideally, the **county seat** is situated in the center of the county, equidistant to all citizens of the county. A centralized easily accessible **county seat** provides equal access to the services there. However, that is not always the case; many counties do not have centrally located **county seats**. Look at the two county maps next.

In the first example of Lenoir County, we see that the **County Seat** (Kinston) is situated in the middle of the county. Citizens throughout the county have almost equal access to the services in the county seat. Compare that with Hyde County, where the **County Seat** of Swan Quarter is situated in the lower quadrant of the county, far away from northern county citizens and difficult to reach by citizens in the northeast corner of the county. For these

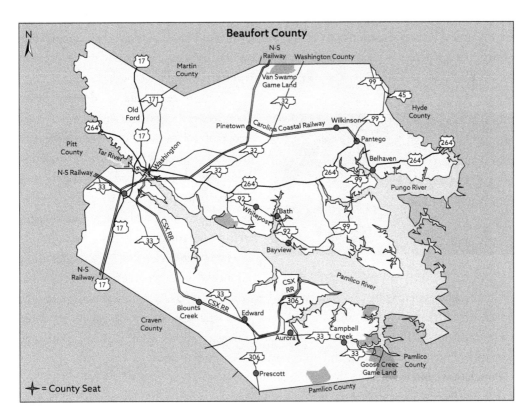

FIGURE 2.3   Beaufort County Map.

rural populations, being unable to reach the county seat equates to having less access to many health and social services.

As important as the county seat may be, the distribution of citizens throughout the county is equally important. Of key interest in health care is not only the actual number of people in an area but also how heavily populated an area is—the **population density**. For instance, we know that in the United States there were roughly 329.2 million as of 2019 (Worldometers, 2019) and that the population density of the United States in that same year was 93 people per square mile (Statista, 2019, *Population density of the U.S.*). By comparison, the state of

APPLICATION OPPORTUNITY

Find the county map for your location. Identify the **county seat** and describe how accessible it might be for citizens in the county.

According to the Census Bureau, **population density** is the number of people per square mile of land area. (U.S. Census Bureau, March 2015; World Population Review, 2019; Worldometers, 2019).

North Carolina had a population of 10.49 million in 2019 (Statisticalatlas, 2019) and a **population density** of 216, whereas in my county the **population density** is approximately 175 persons per square mile (Statista, 2019, *Population density in North Carolina from 1960–2017).*

To measure **population density**, therefore, we need the size in square miles of the geographical unit (e.g., county) and the total number of persons in that unit. **Population density** would be obtained by taking the total number of people living in the county, divided by the square miles in the county, yielding the persons per square mile in the county.

How densely or sparsely populated the county may be provides a data point that is valuable when comparing one county to other counties in the region, when assessing the impact of health interventions, and when looking to see what kind of services might be needed in a physical space. Thus, knowing the population density allows us to plan and ultimately compare interventions, services, and other variables to similar areas.

Population centers consist of towns or communities—they are areas where people live and work. Some federal agencies such as the Census Bureau, describe a minimum number of persons living in an area as the criteria for determining population centers, while some governmental agencies such The North Carolina Office of Budget and Management (NC OBM) use the term "municipalities" as the primary term for **population centers**. For our purposes, we use **population centers** to describe any area in which people live/work, often called towns, townships, municipalities, or communities (NC Budget and Management, Facts and Figures, n.d.).

> **APPLICATION OPPORTUNITY**
>
> Find the **population density** of your state and county. Compare these numbers to the **population density** of the United States and to neighboring states and counties.

> **Population centers** are areas where people live and work, often referred to as towns, townships, municipalities, or cities.

Whatever the term, identifying **population centers** is an important component of assessing and delivering health services. Let us look at two counties with differing **population center** patterns. Craven County has a population of 103,503, and Brunswick County has a relatively similar population at 107,431. So they have comparable number of citizens in the county.

Population Centers Craven County	# People in Population Centers	Population Centers Brunswick County	# People in Population Centers
Bridgeton	454	Bald Head Island	158

Population Centers Craven County	# People in Population Centers	Population Centers Brunswick County	# People in Population Centers
Cove City	399	Belville	1,936
Dover	401	Boiling Springs lake	5,372
Havelock	20,735	Bolivia	143
Newbern	29,524	Calabash	1,786
River Bend	3,119	Carolina Shores	3,048
Trent Woods	4,155	Caswell Beach	398
Vanceboro	1,005	Holden Beach	575
		Leland	13,527
		Navassa	1,505
		Northwest	735
		Oak Island	6,783
		Ocean Island Beach	550
		Sandy Creek	260
		Shallotte	3,675
		Southport	2,833
		St. James	3,165
		Sunset Beach	3,572
		Varnamtown	541
	Total 59,792		Total 50,562

Data from NC Budget and Management, Facts and Figures, n.d.

In Brunswick County, we see that there are 19 **population centers,** with some having few residents. These **population centers** are distributed throughout the county in a relative even distribution with a total of 50,562 people living in population centers. Craven County has a different distribution, eight **population centers** with larger number of people for a total of

APPLICATION OPPORTUNITY

Assume that you wanted to design a program to provide asthma screening to citizens of the two counties listed above, Craven and Brunswick. A specially designed mobile van has been equipped to assess and collect specimens. Think about the resources needed to run the van in each county.

APPLICATION OPPORTUNITY

Using your county, assume that a physician located in the **county seat** wants to open afternoon satellite clinics to treat seasonal ailments. Where would the satellite clinics be placed, and why in that particular location?

59,792 living in these population centers. (NC Budget and Management, Facts and Figures, n.d.). Again, the population is relatively similar in terms of distribution of centers throughout the county, but Craven has more people that can be reached in half as many **population centers**. In planning the delivery of a health care service (see application opportunity) the placement and density of the **population centers** has a direct bearing on resource allocation, design strategies, and implementation feasibility.

Section Review

Thus far we have reviewed that there are four key components within the location element: description of the **topography** of the county, **county seat**, **population density** within the county, and **population centers**. The issue of location is key if the goal is equitable health outcomes for all citizens. We know that citizens in rural communities are located further from health services, while urban citizens (even low-income patients) are often in closer proximity to health care resources. When care is delayed, people experience increased emotional distress, their health condition becomes more complicated, the health care costs rise, and the incidence of hospitalization increases. Thus, for rural citizens, access to health care is a function of location as much as other factors (Office of Disease Prevention and Health Promotion, 2019).

Before leaving this section, it is important to note that while assessing the county (its resources and distribution of citizens) is important, no county is totally isolated from its neighbors. The counties surrounding the county under examination should be identified and included in consideration when evaluating how resources in rural areas can be optimized. For example, a county without a hospital can partner with a neighboring county hospital to improve health care access for its residents. Without county-to-county planning, individuals are left on their own in finding appropriate health services. Nor is location separate from other geographical factors. In the next section, we will examine roads and the impact that roads have on health directly and indirectly by making it possible for citizens to access services.

RUNNING CASE

The Wheelers

Location: The family farm is 700 acres, and while there is a physical address for the farmhouse and barnyard, there is no other address or GPS locator within the 700 acres. The land is comprised of 500 acres of woodland, 150 acres of clear cropland, and the remainder meadow strips and paths.

   One hot summer day while walking and scouting a 30-acre field for insects, Fred begins to feel exhausted and thirsty and develops a headache. He realizes he needs water and the ability to cool down. But his water is in the truck, and as he looks around he realizes it is parked by the previous field he scouted near the woods. Making his way slowly back to the truck, he begins to feel weak and decides he should instead use his cell phone to call help. In the process, he contemplates how to give directions so that someone can find him.

LEARNING ASSESSMENT—LOCATION

Take this Learning Assessment, and then compare your responses to the answers provided at the end of the book. You may find there are elements of the geographical factor you would like to review to gain a better understanding.

1. List the four key topics pertaining to location.
2. Select a county, then list three topographical features of the county.
3. Utilizing the selected county in Question 2, select a topographical feature to be considered as part of health care access, and propose potential solutions to overcome or mediate this obstacle to rural health care access.
4. A centrally located county seat has a positive impact on access to services for people living in rural areas.
   a. True
   b. False
5. List services that are typically located within the county seat of any given county.
6. Fill in the blanks: When calculating population density of a rural area, the _____ population of the county is divided by the _____ within the county to determine the number of people per square mile.
7. Write a brief explanation of how the data regarding population density improves planning health care resources allocation in rural areas.
8. When allocating health resources in a rural area, which of the following county examples would require the most consideration when planning equitable distribution of services?
   a. The county with populations centers located in one region of the county
   b. The county with population centers evenly dispersed across the county

Roads as an Element of the Geographical Factor

This section discusses **Roads** as one of the five elements comprising the geographical factor. We will explore the distinguishing characteristics of rural roads and how they translate to health care issues for people living in rural areas. Think of rural roads you have traveled; remember what they were like. Most of us would recall that rural roads have common characteristics, such as being narrow or bordered by overgrown vegetation. Rural roads are often shared with livestock, wildlife, and large farm equipment. The road surface may be in need of repair, with potholes and cracking. All these characteristics contribute to vehicular accidents or impact the response time of emergency services. In this chapter, we will review the road design features, road shoulders, obstacles, nature of rural road accidents, and EMS response concerns. Collectively, these topics inform the geographical factor element of *roads*.

DESIGN OF RURAL ROADS

We know rural roads were not laid out as part of a master plan to best accommodate modern people traveling in rural areas and are, in fact, poorly suited for modern traffic. That is because rural roads have their beginnings as pathways between neighboring towns and villages. As they walked on foot or rode in wagons pulled by mules, horses, or oxen, early travelers (farmers, trappers, traders) carved out paths. The paths that were created followed whatever contours the traveler or animals found easiest, sometimes between trees, other times meandering along cliffs. Areas near creeks were popular pathways as they provided both direction and a source of water for travelers—human and animal. Understanding how properties were divided helped to ensure that travelers only ventured across friendly areas. Wooded areas with wind breaks in vegetation became easy paths to travel. When it came to crossing water, pragmatic travelers sought low-water crossings at rivers that could be forded easily or that had friendly individuals living at river dwellings who were willing to ferry travelers to the other bank. Again, opportunity and convenience dictated the path.

As a result, the ensuing rural roads were established by the route that was easiest to travel, provided the best footing, stayed dry most the year or provided easy water crossing, and provided the shortest route, given the constraints of the topography and the accessibility of the area. Not surprisingly, given these limitations, roads were often only a single lane that left travelers meeting one another with the decision of who was best positioned to pull to the side so the other could pass. Against this backdrop, the current rural road system has been built. Eventually the dirt roads became paved roads—what we refer to as secondary roads in rural areas—retaining some of their earlier characteristics.

Historically, rural roads have been *narrow* with two lanes of opposing traffic. The standard width of a secondary road is 24 feet (U.S. Department of Transportation, 1993). That is not much room, especially if you consider that an average American pickup is 5 feet wide. That leaves only 3.5 feet on either side of the pickup. It is not hard to understand how a distracted driver can easily swerve a few feet into the path of the oncoming car. The narrowness of rural roads is particularly problematic because roads are shared by a variety of industrial equipment, including farm equipment. We shall return to farm equipment shortly.

> A **secondary road** is a road supplementing a main road, usually wide enough and suitable for two-way, all-weather traffic at moderate or slow speeds (Dictionary of Military and Associated Terms, 2005).

Not only are roads narrow, but rural roads are *curvy*. The curves become accident hazards when drivers under-appreciate the dangers associated with the curve—failing to slow their speed to safely navigate the road's curve, and flying off the curve—or when drivers cannot see what lies beyond the curve—another car or an obstacle (Driving Tips, n.d.). We shall discuss obstacles in the road further into this section, but for now, let us remember that the design of the roads (curvy, narrow) significantly contribute to vehicular accidents and slow rescue travel.

Paved rural roads are not well maintained; some are even gravel roads that have never been paved. This lack of maintenance is evident in *potholes* and cracked road surfaces, missing or damaged road signs, and overgrown vegetation (U.S. Department of Transportation, 2018). We understand how damaged road surfaces and potholes can cause drivers to lose control of their vehicle and have an accident. More problematic is when the damaged or cracked road surface is near the edge of the road, particularly because of the narrow dirt shoulder that we will discuss below. But maintenance issues do not stop with the road surface. Signs on rural roads that caution drivers of upcoming curves or road work, as well as signs indicating location (e.g., highway markers) are sparse, damaged, or missing. Missing or damaged caution signs can contribute to an accident by failing to provide the driver with sufficient warning to slow down for a curve (Driving Tips, n.d.). Lack of signs is also evident near train tracks. In some rural areas, motorists come upon the railroad crossing without any cautionary signal lights or automatic crossing gates to alert them that a train is approaching. Instead, it is expected that rural drivers will be alert enough to check for an oncoming train before crossing a track. Even if vigilant, lack of clear visibility due to overgrown grasses and weeds as well as poor twilight visibility can prevent the driver from easily seeing oncoming trains (Caller Times, 2016).

Another characteristic of rural roads is the *lack of lighting* and *lack of consistent cell phone service*. Rural roads rarely have highway lights or enough ambient light to help drivers navigate the road (Traffic Safety Facts 2017 Data, 2019). This lack of lighting makes it more difficult for a driver to see and to be seen. Take, for instance, a simple task such as changing a flat tire. Even if the driver pulls off the road, changing a flat tire leaves the driver and disabled vehicle in danger because other drivers may not see them stopped on the side of the road. And should the driver want to call a tow truck for assistance with that flat tire, there is poor or no cell service on many stretches of rural roads. The lack of cell reception and lighting not only prevents a tow truck from coming to assist, these same issues can delay first responders from quickly coming to assistance and may, in fact, contribute to a higher mortality rates among rural persons in need.

In addition to lack of maintenance on rural road surfaces, the surrounding area is also poorly maintained (Congressional Research Service, 2018). Rural roads are often lined with vegetation. It is not unusual to see trees close enough to the edge of a road that limbs overhang the road and block visibility, or worse fall onto the road's surface and create physical barriers on the road. Farms have livestock that may escape their fences (e.g., cows) and enter the road, crossing the path of a driver. Wildlife, such as deer, roams rural areas and frequently steps into the road, either directly colliding with a car or causing the driver to swerve and lose control of the vehicle.

ROAD SHOULDERS

Equally as important as the actual design of the road is the lack of **paved shoulders** as a major contributing factor to vehicular accidents and fatalities on rural roads as compared to urban roads. What is a **paved shoulder**, and why is it important? First, the **paved shoulder** is the area surrounding the road that provides the driver with a safe space to pull over off the road for car malfunctions or many other reasons (U.S. Department of Transportation Federal Highway Administration, 1990). The **paved shoulder** allows a margin of safety should a driver inadvertently swerve out of the driving lane, need to correct quickly, or need extra space to correct driving error. In this instance, the **paved shoulder** gives drivers the opportunity to adjust their path before losing control of the vehicle. The **paved shoulder** also serves as an emergency lane used by first responders to access an accident site.

> A **paved shoulder** is constructed of the same material as the road surface. The **paved shoulder** can be as wide as one traffic lane, but at a minimum two to three feet wide.

Unfortunately, most rural roads do not have **paved shoulders**. Take a drive on a rural road and look at what lies beyond the white line. Notice the narrow dirt shoulder—not **paved shoulder**—that drops off below the road's surface. Dirt shoulders are problematic. For one, dirt shoulders do not provide good traction. Driving through a dirt shoulder makes steering a vehicle back onto the road more challenging as wheels may spin and not get sufficient traction to respond quickly. Not only that, but the dirt shoulder—which is often narrow as well unpaved—frequently contains obstacles such as rural mailboxes on posts and road signs that become points of contact if drivers need to leave the road and use the shoulder.

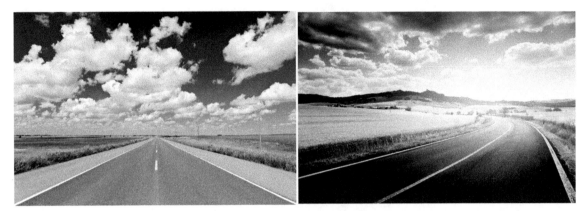

FIGURE 2.4   Road With (left) and Without (right) Paved Shoulder.

Continuing to look at the rural road picture the follows, the next feature we see beyond the shoulder is the ditch. So if the driver needs to correct, driving onto the dirt shoulder often results in driving into the ditch. And the ditch is not devoid of material. Frequently, obstacles like utility poles run the length of the ditch, debris collects in the ditch, and, depending on the time of year, water may fill the ditch. So not only are lack of paved shoulders a safety issue, obstacles in the path of driver on or near the shoulder further increase vehicular impediments.

When accidents occur, the lack of paved shoulders and the narrowness of the shoulder make it difficult for EMS to access an accident scene. In areas with paved shoulders, for example, the shoulders provide a de facto emergency lane, allowing traffic to move off the road so that enable emergency vehicles can either use the main road or bypass traffic by using the shoulder. Instead, with narrow shoulders of dirt, cars cannot safely move aside and rescue vehicles cannot navigate the shoulders well enough to reach their destination. Thus, lack of well paved, sufficient shoulders results in delayed arrival of needed medical care.

OBSTACLES IN THE ROAD

Rural drivers share their rural roads. The overgrown vegetation mentioned above gives cover to wildlife (i.e., deer, elk, and bear) that can spring from their hiding places and run across the roads. The report of 300,000 wildlife–vehicle collisions has been constant for many years (Samsara, 2019). The majority of these collisions involve deer, and nearly 80% of collisions occur in two-lane roads with little traffic. Wildlife is not the only animal obstacle on the road. Animal-related accidents also involve livestock such as cows, horses, or pigs. These animals escape their enclosures and find themselves in the midst of rural traffic.

In addition to animals presenting obstacles for rural drivers, in farming areas, roads are shared with big farm equipment. The average farm tractor is between 9 to 15 feet wide and travels at a speed of 20 miles per hour while towing farming implement that is often wider

APPLICATION OPPORTUNITY

It is dawn and time to plant corn. John is on the road from the barnyard to the field driving a tractor that is pulling a corn planter. Consider the concepts discussed in the previous paragraphs, and apply them to answer these questions.
How does the farm equipment described above maneuver the narrow road and avoid hitting mailboxes and road signs?
How does this maneuver affect vehicles coming up behind the farm equipment and vehicles meeting the farm equipment?
What dangers might exist for the farmworker?
What dangers might exist for drivers of the vehicles?
Watch this YouTube video "Growing Safely—Rural Road Safety": https://www.youtube.com/watch?v=hLYNDTnUTtE
After watching the video, think of three safety measures you can practice while driving on rural roads.

than the tractor. An example of a farming implement is a six-row planter that can be 18 to 20 feet wide. This is a large obstacle on narrow rural roads.

And the time of day that farm equipment is on the road—at dawn when farmworkers are going to the fields and at dusk when returning from the fields—coincides with the time of day that rural commuters are driving to their jobs or returning home. This places commuters anxious to arrive at work or eager to return home on the road at the same time as oversized, slow-moving farm equipment. While it is hard to miss the farm equipment (unless screened by a curve), drivers often misjudge the time it takes them to come upon the farm equipment or miscalculate the actual size of the farm equipment, especially when there is an extended tractor attached to the farm equipment. One study reported that impatient drivers, more than unsafe farm equipment, were the primary culprits for vehicular accidents involving farm equipment.

VEHICULAR ACCIDENTS

Rural roads are not safe. Data provided by the National Highway Traffic Safety Administration reports that more than 50% of all vehicular crashes occur on rural roads, even though there are fewer drivers on these roads and total driving time is less on rural roads. Further breakdown of these statistics shows that about a third of these accidents occur on rural curves and that a higher than normal rate of head-on collisions occur on rural roads. And the results of vehicle accidents are worse for rural drivers. The National Highway Traffic Safety Administration show that drivers on rural roads die at a rate 2.5 times higher per mile traveled than on urban highways (National Public Radio, n.d.).

EMS RESPONSE

When accidents do occur on rural roads, EMS response rates in rural areas are longer than in non-rural areas, both in terms of reaching the patient and transporting to the health care facility. This is one reason that rural drivers in a vehicular accident are more likely to die en route to the hospital than urban drivers (Henning-Smith & Kozhimannil, 2018). For one thing, we know that damaged or missing signage can result in a delay of receiving care. An injured person may not be able to provide sufficient directions to guide rescue workers, and EMS personnel may be unable to locate the scene of an accident with GPS.

Of particular significance is the fact that rural EMS personnel are often volunteers. This means that rescue personnel are most likely occupied when they get a call and must leave their work/family/pastime activities to respond to the emergency call. By some estimates, almost 30% of states depend heavily on some type of volunteer response and volunteer EMS personnel (sometimes by as much as 50%). In some rural areas with low population density, that volunteer figure may go up to as high as 90% volunteer staff. And recruiting new volunteers is challenging. With rural workers required to travel further from home to get jobs, the availability of volunteers to staff rescue in a timely fashion continues to decrease, leaving those that still do the job with an increased workload (National Rural Health Association, n.d.).

CORRIDORS OF DISEASE

We cannot leave our discussion of roads without a few words about the effects that travelers have on relatively isolated and interconnected populations living in small towns. It is often believed that major highways crossing through rural areas can serve as corridors for disease transmission (Forbes, July 2, 2020). People in rural areas who eat at a diner just off a major highway, such as I-95, come in contact with travelers from Maine to Florida. These travelers may spread influenza and communicable diseases not normally appearing in a homogeneous small-town population. Agricultural products are transported by freight trucks and spread bacteria, viruses, and pests that cause illness.

Section Review

We have considered all the characteristics of rural roads and how these characteristics have a direct or indirect impact on the health of people living in rural areas. Fatality data from 2017 shows there were twice the MVA fatalities on rural roads in comparison to urban roads. Rural roads are narrow, curvy, poorly maintained, with no shoulders and overgrown vegetation. These characteristics increase the likelihood of an accident. The lack of signage, GPS, and the distance results in a delay in receiving treatment for injuries and increases the fatality rate. The intensity and the occurrence of accidents are increased due to obstacles such as farm equipment, animals, ditches, utility poles, and mailboxes. Roads used by travelers to rural areas are also corridors for disease transmission.

LEARNING ASSESSMENT—ROADS

Take this Learning Assessment and then compare your responses to the answers provided at the end of the book. You may find there are elements of the geographical factor you would like to review to gain a better understanding.

RUNNING CASE

The Wheelers

Most days Alice does not mind the commute to work. A naturally early riser, Alice leaves home around 6:45 to have plenty of time to get to work. Leaving that early allows her to avoid the school buses or harvest equipment in the fall and planting machinery in the spring. The only problem with leaving that early in the spring is the early morning fog, like this morning. Alice had to go a lot slower in the fog so that 30 minutes into the trip she had not yet passed the open fields and woods. Squinting through the fog, Alice saw a big deer shoot out of the fields just in front of her car. Fearing another deer, Alice slammed on her brakes but not soon enough to avoid colliding with the second deer that crashed into her right front bumper. The collision caused the car to spin and land with its back wheels in the ditch that ran alongside the road. Fortunately, the car stayed upright. "Darn, no bars," bemoaned Alice as she looked at her cell phone and massaged the bump that was forming on her forehead. "I'll just have to wait until someone comes along, maybe that ole school bus will be early today."

1. Rural roads are narrow. Describe how the physical characteristic of being narrow contributes to accidents and injuries on rural roads.
2. Rural roads do not have paved shoulders. Describe how the lack of paved shoulders contributes to accidents and injuries on rural roads and to a delay in EMS arriving at accident sites.
3. Rural roads have overgrown vegetation. Describe how the presence of overgrown vegetation contributes to accidents and injuries on rural roads.
4. Rural roads have more curves than urban roads. Describe how this physical characteristic of being curvier contributes to accidents and injuries on rural roads.
5. Rural areas experience a lack of reliable GPS signal. Describe how the lack of reliable GPS signal can result in a delay in receiving needed medical care.
6. Rural roads have missing or damage signage. Describe how damaged or missing signs can result in a delay in receiving needed medical care.

7. Many obstacles may be present on rural roads. Describe three obstacles and how they might cause an accident.

8. Provide an example of how highways traversing rural roads can be corridors for disease transmission.

9. Visibility on rural roads is diminished at night due to the lack of lighting along the roadway.

    a. True

    b. False

10. Rural roads are safer than urban roads.

    a. True

    b. False

Air as an Element of the Geographical Factor

In this section we will learn about how the characteristic of air in rural areas impacts health. Looking to the available research about the health risks associated with air pollution, we find an abundance of studies conducted in urban settings and less often research specific to rural areas. There is growing recognition of the need for more research examining the health issues related to air pollution in rural areas. There is particular interest in research to understand the significance of location density related to pollution sources such as coal mining and animal operations. Overall, we do know that rural areas have many more pollution sources than urban areas. In this section, there are two key concepts to explore: the sources of air pollution and the impact of unobstructed airflow. We will examine five sources of air pollution and related health issues found in rural populations: forest fires, concentrated animal feeding operations (CAFOs), dust from mining and farming, chemical crop application, and the abundance of pollen.

Rural areas are without physical barriers that obstruct the free flow of air. Knowing air in rural areas flows freely and unobstructed, we can understand that contaminants and **particulate matter** in the air travel wide distances and affect people in more locations over a broader area. In contrast, imagine yourself standing in an urban residential area or a commercial area. What

> **Particulate matter** contains microscopic solids and/or liquid droplets that can be inhaled and cause health problems. These particles can travel into lungs and enter the bloodstream. The particles can be composed of debris from insects and animals, dust, soot, and chemicals.

would you see as you observe your surroundings? Would you see multistoried buildings, privacy fences, and houses lining streets in neighborhoods? These structures in urban areas are close together, providing windbreaks that restrict airflow and impede the spread of air pollution.

> **Unobstructed airflow** occurs when there are no obstacles present to block the wind. For example, a natural windbreak is created by trees, and a manmade windbreak can be created by a building.

Windbreaks slow wind speed by 20% to 30% compared to the **unobstructed airflow** in rural areas. (Encyclopedia Britannica, Urban Climate, 1998).

Let's begin with forest fires as a source of air pollution in rural areas. Eastern North Carolina provides two well-documented examples. The first example occurred in 2008 within the Pocosin Lakes National Wildlife Refuge; another occurred in 2011 in the Alligator River National Wildlife Refuge. Both fires were thought to be caused by lightning. Dry conditions of the forest and the peat-dense forest floor provided fuel, causing the fires to smolder for months. The smoke created by the smoldering peat traveled east to the coast of North Carolina, north into Virginia, and west to Raleigh. People living in this region complained about smelling smoke and seeing a dense haze. Roads were closed at times of low visibility. Exposure to the forest fire smoke resulted in health issues. A of study of 28 counties found an increase in emergency department visits for both cardiac and respiratory conditions (Tinling, 2016).

Another source of air pollution in rural areas is the presence of concentrated animal feeding operations (CAFOs). The **CAFOs** are large low-built structures where the animals are confined.

> **CAFOs** stands for **concentrated animal feeding operations**. **CAFOs** are agricultural enterprises that feed and raise animals in confined spaces.

The animals eat, sleep, urinate, and defecate in these spaces, creating airborne effluent. **CAFOs** are utilized for cattle, hogs, chickens, or turkeys. They are typically found in rural areas where land is less expensive, creating the situation where **CAFOs** are located in areas where our poorest populations live. Also, lower land prices often dictate where schools are built, thus placing **CAFOs** and schools in close proximity to one another. In the example of swine operations, the liquid and solid waste is flushed from the confined space into open-air lagoons (U.S. Department of Agriculture, n.d.). The water from the lagoons is then sprayed onto fields. Chicken or turkey operations can have thousands of animals whose waste accumulates on the floors of the structures. Their waste is collected at intervals and loaded into spreader trucks. The spreader trucks spread the dry waste material onto fields (U.S. Department of Agriculture, n.d.). Some of the air pollutants from swine and poultry operations are ammonia, hydrogen sulfide, methane, bacteria, fungi, and endotoxins. The health effects for people working in the **CAFOs** or living within proximity are increased incidence of respiratory problems, specifically asthma. The odors from **CAFOs** cause mental health concerns such as depression. Other reported health issues are headaches, migraines, runny nose, sore throat, excessive coughing, diarrhea, and burning eyes (Loftus, et al., 2015).

Farming and mining activities generate their own kinds of dust. This dust becomes part of the air that people living and working in rural areas breathe. In farming the dust generated by farming may be called agricultural dust or respirable **organic dust**.

But whatever the name, we know the air in rural areas contains a mixture of particulate matter that is composed of animal dander, insect parts, chemical residue, molds, and fungi.

> **Organic dust** is dust with particulate matter that is biologically active and capable of causing respiratory tract responses that can be allergic, inflammatory, toxic, or infectious.

TABLE 2.1 Agents and Common Names for Hypersensitivity Pneumonitis (HP) Among Agricultural Workers and Food Product Processors.

Exposure	Agent[1]	Common Name or Condition
Moldy hay or silage	*Thermophilic actinomycetes* *Micropolyspora faeni* Others	Farmer's Lung
Mushroom production/ mushroom compost	*Thermoactinomycetes vulgaris* Others	Mushroom Worker's Lung
Moldy sugar cane plant residue—post processing	*S. viridis* *T. sacchari* Others	Bagassosis
Fungi		
Moldy maple bark	*Cryptostroma corticale* Others	Maple Bark Stripper's Disease
Moldy malt	*Aspergillus clavatus* Others	Malt Worker's Lung
Moldy cork dust	*Penicillium frequentans* Others	Suberosis
Surface mold on cheese	*P. caseii* Others	Cheese Worker's Lung
Moldy wood chips	*Altervaria spp.* Others	Wood Worker's Lung People using wood chips for heating fuel

---

1 *Note.* There likely are multiple agents of hypersensitivity pneumonitis for each specific condition. Specific agents listed here have been associated with the condition but are probably just one of several agents involved.

TABLE 2.1   Agents and Common Names for Hypersensitivity Pneumonitis (HP) Among Agricultural Workers and Food Product Processors. (*continued*)

Exposure	Agent[1]	Common Name or Condition
Moldy redwood dust	*Pullularia spp.* Others	Sequoiosis
Paprika dust	*Mucor spp.* Others	Paprika Splitter's Lung
Arthropods		
Infested wheat	*Sitophilus granarius* Others	Wheat Weevil Disease
Fresh avian droppings	Avian proteins	Bird Breeder's Lung

Source: Kelley J. Donham and Anders Thelin, "Agents and Common Names for Hypersensitivity Pneumonitis (HP) among Agricultural Workers and Food Product Processors," *Agricultural Medicine: Occupational and Environmental Health for the Health Professions*, p. 83. Copyright © 2016 by Blackwell Publishing.

The activities of farming create and disperse **organic dust**. Some examples include harvesting or storing grains, opening bales of molded hay, plowing fields, and managing livestock. The health effect is dependent on the type of exposure, the duration, the intensity, and the baseline health of the individual exposed. Farmers and farmworkers are most directly affected, as are their families (U.S. Department of Labor, n.d.). The particulate matter is transported into the homes and living spaces of their families on their clothing when they return from work.

The dust from coal mining is a source of pollution in rural areas. Using West Virginia as our example, there are air monitoring stations located around the state, but none of the monitoring stations are located in areas that are primarily coal mining communities. However, research demonstrates that coal mining is a risk factor for higher mortality rates from cancer and respiratory illnesses (Hendryx et al., 2010). We see fields or mines surrounding houses as we drive through rural areas. Many of these houses are occupied by families that are not connected with farming or mining. Yet, by living in the rural area, they are exposed to air pollution generated by farming and mining activities.

Chemical crop application is a source of air pollution in rural areas. Spraying or dustings are common methods used to apply chemicals to field crops. The chemical application is accomplished by planes that fly over fields or by tractors that are driven through the fields. The spraying application is a fine water mist containing chemicals. The dusting application is a fine, dry granular material. Both forms are easily carried through the air to places other than the intended crops (Arcury et al., 2014). So farm chemicals are sources of air pollution, but air pollution is also created by farm equipment. Let's consider the example of a farmer driving a tractor through a field fumigating the soil in preparation for planting strawberries. The farmer will drive this diesel-fueled tractor for 8 to 10 hours a day, inhaling diesel exhaust. The field in which the farmer is driving his tractor has been tilled and therefore creates a lot of dust as the tractor moves through the field. The dust in the air contains organic particulate matter described earlier. The fumigant being applied to the soil is carried on the air and can be inhaled as well as easily absorbed through skin contact. Chemical exposures have negative health effects, including various types of cancers—multiple myeloma, non-Hodgkin's lymphoma, prostate cancer, and breast cancer. Agricultural chemical exposures are also associated with Parkinson's disease and dementia (Owens et al., 2010).

Pollen is abundant in rural areas due to heavy vegetation. There are more trees, weeds, grasses, and crops than in urban areas. Spring and fall are two seasons when the pollen is especially thick, and the long-needle pine provides its share of pollen in eastern North Carolina. While pollen is essential for plants to propagate and grow, it causes a long list of allergy-related illnesses including asthma, rhinitis, and sinusitis.

Rural populations live in closer proximity to types of vegetation that generate a generous amount of pollen. This, along with a greater diversity in variety of pollen-producing plants, makes rural pollen exposure higher for people living in rural areas.

Section Review

Rural health can be positively impacted by awareness of the health issues associated with air pollution in rural areas. Policies to decrease or mediate air pollution can be better informed with the placement of air monitors near pollution sources. Planning in rural communities is enhanced by recognizing the health concerns associated with placement of **CAFOs** in close proximity to schools. Similarly, planning could avoid placing several mines in close proximity and creating dense air-pollution areas. For better health outcomes, providers must understand the potential airborne threats that exist in their rural practice area so that they may better diagnose and treat rural populations.

> ### APPLICATION OPPORTUNITY
>
> The American Academy of Allergy Asthma and Immunology provides information and education about health effects. An interactive map provides actual pollen and mold counts for specific cities. Find your location and explore the pollen count as well as health issues related to pollen exposure. https://www.aaaai.org/global/nab-pollen-counts?ipb=1

RUNNING CASE

The Wheelers

Air: The August air was just stifling with high temperatures and little rain. Fortunately, there was some air movement. But that was not all good. The ground was beginning to look parched, and everywhere anyone walked or drove stirred up dust that was easily carried through the air. This was particularly noticeable on the soccer field at the high school. The varsity team had begun practice 2 weeks earlier in anticipation of its first game when school started. Early morning practice was OK, but late afternoon practice was really bad—dust seemed to float around everywhere. If that wasn't bad enough, the kids' allergies were acting up as roadside ragweed began blooming. The coach had his hands full with dust, ragweed, and sweaty high school boys running laps around the pitch.

LEARNING ASSESSMENT—AIR

Take this Learning Assessment and then compare your responses to the answers provided at the end of the book. You may find there are elements of the geographical factor you would like to review to gain a better understanding.

1. List five sources of air pollution in rural areas.
2. Rural areas have restricted airflow due to physical obstacles that create windbreaks.
   a. True
   b. False
3. List two health issues that are associated with exposure to smoke from forest fires.
4. List four health issues related to exposure to pollution from CAFOs.
5. Organic dust is particulate matter that is biologically active and capable of causing respiratory tract illnesses.
   a. True
   b. False
6. Air pollution in rural areas is more varied in its makeup and travels further than air pollution in urban areas.
   a. True
   b. False
7. Describe two common methods for applying chemicals to crops.
8. People living in rural areas and not associated with farming have no risk exposure to agricultural chemicals.
   a. True
   b. False

9. List three health issues relate to pollen exposure.
10. Pollen exposure is higher for people living in rural areas compared to people living in urban areas.

Water as an Element of the Geographical Factor

We all know that water benefits us directly and indirectly. We need water to drink and to feed our plants. Livestock need water to survive, and we fish in water. Water also provides us transportation and recreation. But water can directly and indirectly cause health concerns, and these health concerns differ in urban and rural areas. In this section, we explore rural water and its impact on health. Along the way, we will explore how rural populations obtain **drinking water**; issues related to rural excess water, normally in the form of **runoff**; standing water leading to **vector-borne diseases**; and rural water used for **recreational and transportation** purposes. In each section, we will explore the health concerns associated with these four water matters.

DRINKING WATER

Drinking water sources often differ for urban and rural populations. According to EPA, more than 90% of Americans get their drinking water from public water systems (CDC, 2020). These are the systems whereby a municipality collects water, ensures its safety for distribution, and then distributes the water through a series of pipes from its point of collection to home faucets throughout its service areas.

Public water systems are the sole drinking water distribution system in urban areas. In rural areas, some citizens receive their drinking water through **public water systems**. Alternatively, some use private wells that are dug to gain access to underground water sources and pumped directly into households for drinking and household use.

Unlike **public water systems**, water obtained through wells has the following unique features:

> **Public water systems** may be privately owned as well as publicly owned. To be called a **public water system** the water must be for human consumption and provide service to an average of at least 25 people per day through at least 15 water connections (U.S. EPA—Information about Public Water Systems).

a. Typically, well water is untreated water, per se. That means that the water is obtained directly from the primary source, the aquifer, and transported directly into homes. Well water does not go through a municipal treatment facility.

b. Well water may or may not contain naturally occurring fluoride. Water normally contains some fluoride that is enhanced when public water systems treat the water to ensure a level of fluoride beneficial to water recipients. However, few private wells are treated with additional fluoride. Thus, it is often noted that water obtained through a private well does not contain sufficient fluoride to ensure benefits such as healthier teeth (KidsHealth from Nemours. April 15, 2015).

c. Well water may contain higher levels of minerals such as calcium, magnesium, and iron that might make the water hard, smelly, or prone to creating rust stains.

d. Well water must be tested periodically to ensure that the water is safe from surface runoff or naturally occurring contaminates such as radon or arsenic (American Ground Water Education, 2018).

Top Six Causes of Outbreaks in Individual (Private) Water Systems (CDC, July 2 2015):

1. Hepatitis A
2. Giardia
3. Campylobacter, *E. coli* (tie)
4. Shigella
5. Cryptosporidium, *Salmonella* (tie)
6. Arsenic, Gasoline, Nitrate, Phenol, Selenium (tie)

Responsibility to test well water and ensure its suitability for drinking resides with the well owner. This is in direct contrast to public water systems where the municipality takes responsibility for carrying out inspections and providing safe water treatment.

To illustrate this difference, let's look at two families. The Jones family lives in a small metropolitan area of 100,000 people. They receive their water through the **public water system**. This water is treated by a municipal treatment plant, tested periodically for a variety of contaminants, and supplied to the Jones's household. The city funds water treatment and distribution through a combination of charges passed on to the Jones (e.g., water usage charges) and municipal and state funds allocated for infrastructure. The Smith household relies on well water. Here the water is obtained from a **private well** found on their property. The Smith family relies on well water both because they feel as if the water tastes better and because the city does not provide water services

> A **private well** is constructed access to groundwater for human consumption and is designed to serve an average of 24 or fewer people per day through 14 or fewer connections (CDC, 2014).

this far into the county. It is the responsibility of the Smith family to periodically inspect the water to ensure sanitation levels are met. No one specifically oversees the Smith's household to ensure that that safety measures are being carried out; it is the responsibility of the well owner to monitor their own drinking water. Keep these two households in mind as we progress through several other concepts. Let's start with excess water, especially in the form of runoff.

RUNOFF WATER

Runoff water can occur from natural weather events (storms, melting rain) or from man-made occurrences (e.g., overwatering lawns or opening levies).

In urban areas, runoff typically occurs because there is insufficient soil to absorb the amount of water being deposited (Climate Central, February 28, 2018). Think city environments with lots of concrete walkways or driveways, paved streets, and blocks of parking lots. There is often no place for the water to be absorbed so it creates urban runoff that carries petroleum products (gasoline, oil, etc.) normally found in its path along city streets and driveways.

Rural **runoff water** is different. Here there is soil to absorb the water, but sometimes the amount of water is too great for the soil to absorb. So rural runoff flows over soil, while traveling through open fields, wooded areas, mining sites, and agricultural areas. As such, rural runoff is more likely to carry products found in the soil—pesticides or fertilizers as nutrient pollution when it travels through farming communities (Theodore Roosevelt Conservation Partnership, November 9, 2017) or acid mine drainage when to goes through mining communities (Earthworks, n.d.). That is not to say that some urban runoff does not find its way into rural areas (often

---

APPLICATION OPPORTUNITY

Is there an extra burden placed on the Smith household because they rely on private well water? If so, how can this burden be lessened?

Runoff water occurs at times when there is more water present than the ground can absorb. The excess water runs along the surface of the ground until it is eventually absorbed or enters a body of water. As the water travels the ground's surface, it collects and carries chemicals and debris that it comes in contact with along the way.

APPLICATION OPPORTUNITY

Consider the effects of **runoff water** to the Jones's and Smith's households. How might runoff impact drinking water in each household? Who would be responsible for treating the **runoff water** prior to having the household consume the water?

through downstream impacts), but for the most part rural area runoff is a product of the material found in the surrounding open areas.

Runoff is made more problematic when it leads to standing water or an increase in the amount of water in ponds, creeks, or smaller water settings. Either of these scenarios gives rise to increases in vector-borne diseases. We are all familiar with the mosquito, one of the most prolific vectors to afflict us. Other vectors include ticks and fleas. In rural areas where there is much water, these vectors multiply.

VECTOR-BORNE DISEASES

Some of the most common vector-borne diseases according to the U.S. Global Change Research program are Lyme disease, transmitted by ticks, and West Nile virus, transmitted by mosquitoes (n.d.). Many areas have seen a rise in the prevalence of these diseases, but their rate is not equal. For instance, North Carolina trends show that the rise has been in the tick-borne illnesses, rather than mosquito-borne illnesses, as shown in Figure 2.5 (CDC, 2019).

So while mosquitoes might be a greater nuisance, ticks result in greater health concerns.

APPLICATION OPPORTUNITY

Using your home county or your state, look up the type of vector-borne illnesses that are in your area. Determine if there have been changes (increases or decreases) in the type of frequency of vector-borne illnesses.

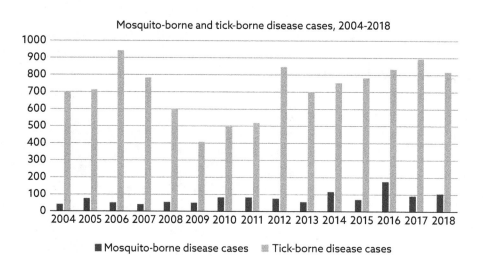

FIGURE 2.5   Mosquito-Borne and Tick-Borne Disease Cases, 2004–2016.

RECREATIONAL ACTIVITIES

Early settlers often depended on rural waterways as primary transportation sources. While that is no longer the case, rural waterways (rivers, lakes, ponds, creeks) provide rural residents with an abundance of recreational opportunities. Residents close to these water sources enjoy swimming, boating, fishing, and playing in and around water. Each of these activities poses a potential health concern, some differing significantly from health risks faced by urban dwellers.

The most serious concern is drowning, often identified as one of the leading causes of death due to unintentional injury in people under 18. Drowning rates for rural residents are as much as three times higher than drowning rates in urban areas.[3] And the settings for drownings are different. In urban settings, drownings most often occur in pools. In rural areas, on the other hand, drownings occur in natural settings such as ponds, lakes, or even irrigation canals. Higher rural drowning rates may be attributable to youths swimming unsupervised or even alone. Moreover, the isolation of the settings makes rescue efforts problematic; a possible drowning may go unnoticed or not be responded to in a timely fashion.[4]

Other recreational health concerns include boating accidents (a relatively small

Vector-borne disease cases

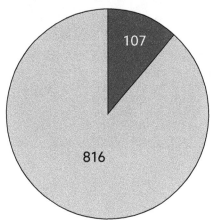

- ■ Mosquito-borne disease cases
- ☐ Tick-borne disease cases

FIGURE 2.6   Tick Vector-Borne Disease Cases.

In its simplest definition, **standing water** is any form of water that does not flow or move.

Vectors transmit diseases between humans or from animals to humans. Vectors are living organisms, such as ticks and mosquitoes.[2]

---

2   World Health Organization. (October 31, 2017).

3   National Ag Safety Database. (n.d.). Rural water safety. Retrieved April 7, 2021: https://nasdonline.org/1858/d001799/rural-water-safety.

4   Yang, L., Nong, Q. Q., Li, C. L., Feng, Q. M., & Lo, S. K. (2007). Risk factors for childhood drowning in rural regions of a developing country: a case-control study. *Injury Prevention : Journal of the International Society for Child and Adolescent Injury Prevention, 13*(3), 178–182. https://doi.org/10.1136/ip.2006.013409

risk factor given the total number of people who enjoy boating), jet ski injuries (often resulting in orthopedic injuries from collisions or inappropriate driving techniques), fishing injuries (such as fish hook punctures or even hypothermia from ice fishing), and various water illnesses associated with water activities.[5] Attentiveness and adherence to safety protocols is critical to mitigate water-related injuries and illnesses.

Section Review

Water is prominent in rural areas. Where residents obtain their drinking water, how runoff occurs and what is carried in the runoff, which vector-borne diseases might affect the area due to standing water, and even recreational health risks differ between rural and urban settings. Each topic helps inform the element of water as a geographical factor that describes and impacts rural health.

RUNNING CASE

The Wheelers

Water: Fred was in the back pasture when he spotted the kids four-wheeling down to the pond. It rained yesterday so he knew that the pond would be full—perfect for early summer swimming. "Be careful of water moccasins," he called out to the kids as they slowed down not far from where he was working. "We know" they yelled back in unison. "And," he began. "We know," interrupted the kids as they drove on past, "check for ticks as soon as we get home." "Yes," said Fred, knowing that the pond was a favorite spot for deer and their fawns as they ventured further out of the woods in the spring.

5   Targett S., & Geertsema C. (2014).

LEARNING ASSESSMENT—WATER

Take this Learning Assessment and then compare your responses to the answers provided at the end of the book. You may find there are elements of the geographical factor you would like to review to gain a better understanding.

1. Private wells are the most common sources of drinking water for people living in rural areas.
   a. True
   b. False
2. List three water-related diseases associated with private wells.
3. The owner of a private well is responsible for testing the water safety.
   a. True
   b. False
4. Provide an example of man-made runoff water.
5. Naturally occurring runoff water in mining communities may contain _____ _____ _____.
6. List two vectors that may be attached to standing water.
7. Select one of the vectors, and identify the disease transmitted by the vector.
8. List three ways that water is beneficial.

Weather as an Element of the Geographical Factor

No one would argue that weather affects health. Long hot summers encourage us to stay outdoors longer, often resulting in our later suffering a serious sunburn. But nice summer weather also encourages us to abandon our socks and heavy shoes to put on sandals, flip-flops, or even go without shoes. The health concerns? Stubbed or broken toes, punctures from stepping barefoot on a myriad of pointy objects (stones, twigs, trash). In this section, we are going to explore three weather/climate concerns—precipitation, flooding, heat-related and cold-related illness.

PRECIPITATION

Precipitation comes in the form of showers, downpours, blizzards, snow flurries, nor 'easters, and hurricanes. Let's look at precipitation in the form of rain. Over the past decade, the number of rainy days (rain frequency) and the accumulations from these

APPLICATION OPPORTUNITY

Of interest is to see how the rain patterns have affected your area. For instance, in our hometown of Greenville, North Carolina, the rain trends are increasing.

Follow this link to look at your state or city to see the changes in rainfall in your area: https://www.climatecentral.org/gallery/graphics/heavy-rainfall-trends-us

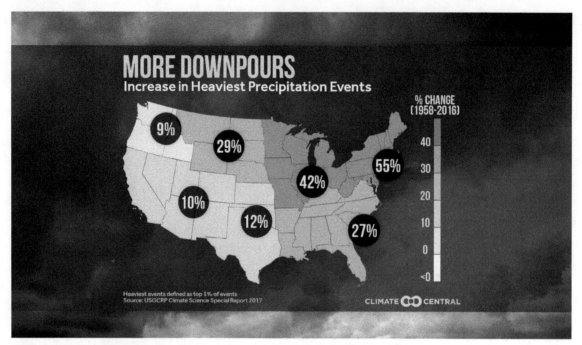

FIGURE 2.7   More Downpours: Increase in Heaviest Precipitation Events.

rainy days has changed. As can be seen in trends publicized by Climate Central,[6] nationally there have been more downpours, especially in some areas of the county.

Increased amounts of rain trigger among other things an increase in water runoff and the corresponding issues we discussed in the previous section. But increase in rain intensity also triggers dry land conditions in rural, agricultural areas. How is that? Well, in its simplest explanation, when it rains a lot water does not have time to be absorbed in the soil and instead travels across the soil surface as runoff. The end result of this rain deluge is that the soil does not have a chance to be saturated, cannot increase the aquifer that feeds the soil so that the soil has no way of retaining sufficient moisture to offset dry days. Then when dry days come, the land dries faster and triggers what we commonly think of as a drought-like condition. As we shall see in the next chapter, farmers are particularly adversely impacted by this cycle of more rainy days, loss of saturation, and dry land conditions.

FLOODING

More intense and frequent rain also triggers another rural concern—flooding. As we mentioned previously, there are a lot of water bodies in rural areas. As rain days and rain accumulations increase, water levels in creeks and rivers increase to the point where they overflow their

---

6   Climate Central. (April 11, 2019).

banks and create flood conditions. Likewise, intense rain also triggers what we commonly call a flash flood condition.

Flooding has direct health concerns. Not only do people drown as floodwater carries them away, but the aftermath of floods is often an increase in mildew and mold. In turn, increase mold triggers increases in respiratory issues (e.g., congestion, wheezing, asthma-like symptoms and coughs), while prolonged proximity to mold might trigger actual asthmatic attacks. (National Capital Poison Center, n.d.). Apart from mold, floodwater might also carry pollutants or waste products that increase wound infections, contact dermatitis (Medical Press, March 1, 2019), and even might trigger gastrointestinal illnesses or tetanus (Centers for Disease Control and Prevention, Sept. 13, 2018). And, flooding does not affect all segments of the population equally. Often the poor and most vulnerable rural populations are most negatively impacted by floods.

A less obvious health concern with flooding is the impact that the flood has on emergency services, including rescue personnel. As we noted earlier, rural roads have inherent hazards and obstacles. These roads are often abutting waterways or constructed in low-lying areas, making them susceptible to frequent flooding. When this occurs, EMS or other rescue personnel have an even more difficult time arriving at their destination. Additionally, rural populations that depend on these roads are often victims in flooded conditions to hydroplaning, without the safety margins of shoulders or guardrails.

> **APPLICATION OPPORTUNITY**
>
> Find rain changes in your area. Identify flood conditions in your region. How have these flood conditions changed over the past 10 years?

HEAT-RELATED ILLNESSES

Another weather topic we should discuss is the change in heat and corresponding rise in **heat-related illness**. Just as rainfall is rising, so is the number of days exceeding 100 °F in temperature (Climate Central, May 16, 2018). In the past 30 years, the average temperature in the United States has risen by 1.4 °F, which translates into more days above 90 degrees. This temperature upsurge has caused an increase in heat-related illness: heat exhaustion, heat stroke, dehydration, heat cramps, heat rash, and skin melanoma (Centers for Disease Control and Prevention, n.d.).

> **Heat-related illness** is also called hyperthermia and occurs with exposure to heat conditions. It means the body's temperature is too high and the body has lost the ability to regulate temperature. Picture of America Heat-Related Illness Fact Sheet (cdc.gov)

Heat-related illnesses are of particular concern in rural areas (as we shall explore further in the next chapter) because so many rural occupations are outdoor jobs: farming, logging, fishing,

APPLICATION OPPORTUNITY

Using the following website, identify your home town and year of birth to see how much hotter your town is now: https://www.nytimes.com/interactive/2018/08/30/climate/how-much-hotter-is-your-hometown.html.

forestry, as well as typical small businesses of construction and landscaping.

Equally as important as occupations that put people at risk for heat-related illness, increase in temperatures (number of days and degrees) also impacts people who live in non-air-conditioned housing, such as temporary migrant housing. Unlike in urban areas where people without home air-conditioning might find refuge from the heat in public spaces (libraries, malls, or community pools), rural areas may lack such public spaces. Thus, there is little relief for rural citizens who do not have air conditioning.

As with water and temperatures, the incidence of fires is increasing. Fire season is lengthening, along with fire intensity. According to the Center for Climate and Energy Solutions,

> **Fire intensity** is the heat energy of the fire (National Park Service/USDA Forest Service, n.d.).

> **Fire Season** is the time the year when forest fires are most likely to occur (National Park Service/USDA Forest Service, n.d.).

today we have more wildfires, hotter fires, and fires that burn larger land masses than we did in the past. Rural areas are prime targets for these fires, especially in dry conditions where lightning strikes might ignite the dry grasses. Equally, as we discussed with airflow, rural areas with few barriers to airflow allow particulates from fires to spread unobstructed through the area.

COLD-RELATED ILLNESSES

Winter weather presents health and safety concerns for rural communities as well. Unlike rainfall changes, the changes in snow days, snow accumulation, and the frequency of snowstorms is less clear. Experts who follow changes in snow and winter patterns seems to agree that the length of the snow season is shorter than it was in the past. Likewise, there is also agreement that when snowstorms do occur, the severity of the storm is greater than in the past (National Snow and Ice Data Center, 2020). While in the next chapter we might want to consider the economic impact of these changes (e.g., the impact of shortened snow seasons on rural communities dependent upon tourism), in this chapter we will focus specifically on the rural health impacts of winter weather. Differences do emerge on how rural populations fare in winter weather.

As in hot weather, the lack of public buildings and businesses in rural areas becomes a hardship in winter. Without this infrastructure, rural people rely solely on their homes for warmth. While there has been significant decline in households using space heaters as primary sources of heat, there are still many households in rural areas that rely on such a heating source (U.S. Energy Information Administration, April 6, 2017; Harrison & Popke, 2011). Individuals using space heaters are at a higher risk for burns, carbon monoxide poisoning, and asphyxiation when houses are not well ventilated. Rural residents without adequate heating suffer from cold-induced ailments such as cold-induced asthma, arthritis, and of course colds, though it is worth mentioning that flu trends have declined since 2012. When snow and ice storms occur, emergency departments see an increase in musculoskeletal injuries resulting from slipping and falling on icy surfaces. Outdoor workers, often prevalent in rural areas, are at risk for these types of illnesses, as well as more serious conditions such as hypothermia and frostbite (Ag Safety and Health, 2021).

Section Review

While changing weather patterns occur indiscriminate of rural–urban distinctions, the means by which the community can deal with these weather changes is very distinct. Rural areas rarely have the infrastructure to deal with changes in weather patterns. Rural areas have fewer resources to curtail or deal with flooding, provide shelters from the heat, or provide services associated with heat- or cold-related illness. As we shall see in the next chapter describing the economic factor, poorer areas suffer disproportionately from weather-related concerns. That is to say, rural areas are more adversely affected by changing weather concerns.

RUNNING CASE

The Wheelers

Weather: September had been a particularly rainy month, and yesterday's storm (the outer ridge of an offshore hurricane) was particularly problematic. The past month's rain had left the grounds saturated so yesterday's rain overwhelmed streams and creeks and turned into flash floods in low-lying areas. Fortunately, the high school band bus (with Evie on it) had made it to the school just in time, but there was no getting into or out of the school. One road was blocked by a fallen tree uprooted in the storm; the other road was completely covered in water. Alice knew that she would have to wait until the water receded to go get Evie. In the meantime, the kids would wait in the cafeteria—a place well equipped to handle local evacuees in times like this.

LEARNING ASSESSMENT—WEATHER

Take this Learning Assessment and then compare your responses to the answers provided at the end of the book. You may find there are elements of the geographical factor you would like to review to gain a better understanding.

1. The number of rainy days has increased in the past decade.
   a. True
   b. False
2. Name four health issues that arise in relation to flooding.
3. Temperatures have decreased over the past several decades.
   a. True
   b. False
4. Another name for heat-related illnesses is _____.
5. Name four heat-related illnesses.
6. Explain how the lack of public spaces impacts heat exposure of people living in rural communities.
7. Select the answer that best exemplifies the cause and effect relationship between weather and health issues.
   a. Flooding promotes mold growth.
   b. Winter ice storms result in fallen trees on roads.
   c. Sun exposure increases the risk of heat stroke.
   d. Winter ice storms make roads slippery, causing an increase in automobile accidents that result in injury.

CHAPTER SUMMARY

In this chapter we reviewed the five elements that comprise the geographical factor: location, roads, air, water, and weather. We drilled down in each element to identify key concepts that explain how the element contributes to health concerns and health outcomes in rural populations. While these elements are significant independent of each other, most often the elements interconnect with each other to form a more profound effect. Thus, it is important to be comprehensive in identifying data for each of the elements in order to collectively produce a complete picture of the rural community.

One way to ensure that we capture all the geographical elements is to complete the Geographical Factor Assessment Grid (see Table 2.2). By answering each of the questions on the grid, no element is excluded or minimized. Instead, the completed grid allows us to efficiently view key characteristics that are known to impact the health of the citizens of that county.

Not only can we use the grid to provide a snapshot of the geographical elements in the county, but we can use the grid to help us explain what we are viewing and even identify missing issues that might help inform us as to the nature of rural health challenges. For practice applying the Geographical Factor County Assessment Grid Template, take the two learner challenges at the end of this chapter.

Just as these elements do not stand alone in their impact on rural health, in the next chapter we shall see how the factors do not stand alone either. We have already begun in this chapter to see how economic factors might impact the ability of the county to build infrastructure to mitigate changes in weather or impacts from adverse weather effects or to build safer roads. Thus, the journey of identifying those issues that impact rural health continues in the next chapter on economic factors.

TABLE 2.2 Geographical Factor County Assessment Grid Template

Factor	Element	County Data	Source & Comments
Geographical	Location	County map—place your county here.	
		Describe topology issues if not evident on map.	
		Population Density	
		Give the square miles in county—population per square mile.	
		County Seat Name and locate the county seat.	
		Describe how central (or not central) the county seat is relative to other population centers.	
		Population Centers	
		Give location of major population centers.	
		Give population numbers for these centers.	
	Roads	Identify roads throughout the county and describe these in terms of primary or secondary roads.	
		Identify any corridors of disease in the county.	
		Describe health statistics relative to roads: Vehicular accidents & fatalities Placement of EMS and response time	

TABLE 2.2   Geographical Factor County Assessment Grid Template *(continued)*

Factor	Element	County Data	Source & Comments
	Air	Describe air quality. For instance, Particulate matter CAFOs Organic dust Pollen	
		Describe airflow and any obstacles to impede air flow.	
		List major air-related health concerns in the county.	
	Water	Locate major bodies of water in the county and describe how they are used (drinking, transportation, recreation, commercial fishing, etc.).	
		Identify vector-borne disease patterns in the county.	
		Describe how most citizens obtain drinking water in the county.	
	Weather	Describe any changes in frequency or intensity of weather issues (heat, rain, fires, snow, etc.).	
		Identify heat- and cold-related illness and any changing patterns in the county.	

CHAPTER ACTIVITY—LEARNING CHALLENGE

Below are two learning challenges designed to help apply the geographical factor's elements in a systematic review. The learning challenges can be completed individually or in small group.

Learning Challenge 1: Using your county or a selected county, complete the Geographical Factor Assessment Grid. Be sure to populate each element with comprehensive data elements. Use visuals (e.g., maps) to supplement the data elements and narrative. Be sure to include all sources from which data was obtained.

Learning Challenge 2: Complete the following scenario using your county or a selected county: Scenario: The State Health and Human Resources Department is considering allocating block grants to improve EMS services at the county level. They have asked you to identify data elements that should be included in a grant application. Your task is to review the Geographical Factor Assessment Grid and

a. Identify which elements are important data to be included in the proposal. Please describe for each element why and how you feel that inclusion of this data element would enhance county planning for EMS services.

  b. Identify which elements in the grid do not need to be included in any county proposal, and describe why that element is not important enough to include.

CHAPTER ACTIVITY—PRACTICE VIGNETTES

Below are three practice vignettes. Read the scenario, and answer the questions following each scenario. These practice vignettes may be completed individually or in small groups.

Vignette 1: The Mackenfield family likes rural life. Mrs. Mackenfield works part time as a cashier at Dollar General. When she is not at work, she takes care of their three children: Toby, age 17; Angie, age 15; and little Bobby, age 7. She plants a large vegetable garden that supplies the family with much of their fresh and canned vegetables and raises prized Malti-Poos (a cross between Maltese and Poodle) in a large dog pen. Mr. Mackenfield is a salesperson in the Rocky Mount Dodge dealership, a job he likes because it allows him to set his own hours. He and his brother cultivate timber on land they inherited from their father. When not working, Mr. Mackenfield can be found fishing or hunting.

  a. Explain why the Mackenfield's are at greater risk for vehicular accidents with resulting injuries and/or fatalities because of where they live.
  b. Mr. Mackenfield likes to hunt. Should he have an accident and need EMS, describe why it would be more difficult for him to obtain medical attention.
  c. Mr. Mackenfield's dealership job is just off I-95. He often eats at a diner frequented by a lot of travelers on I-95. Explain why he might be more at risk for getting diseases from outside the area because of the location of this eatery.

Vignette 2: Jeff is a second grader, 7 years old, who unfortunately suffers from asthma. He attends an elementary school in a rural area. Naturally, Jeff's mom is concerned about sending Jeff to school each day but is comforted by knowing that Jeff has an experienced teacher (Ms. Wellons) who is familiar with asthma triggers and how to obtain help for children like Jeff. From years of being in the classroom, Ms. Wellons knows that there are several times throughout the year where asthma attacks might be exacerbated by environmental factors. The County Health Department provides health education material for teachers relative to asthma and other childhood illnesses, and the school has a nurse assigned to the elementary school. Ms. Wellons uses these resources frequently. Still, Jeff's mom is concerned.

  a. Identify air or water issues in rural areas that could trigger asthma attacks.
  b. Describe why airflow in rural areas is different than airflow in urban areas and how this difference can increase the likelihood of Jeff experiencing respiratory problems.

    c. In addition to asthma, what other health conditions might be triggered from airborne pathogens in rural areas?

    d. Explain why the location of the county seat, which may include resources such as the County Health Department, impacts the health care access of Jeff and the other students at the rural elementary school.

Vignette 3: Every year a rural island community prepares for its summer visitors. These visitors are the economic lifeblood of the island and help support its 900+ year-round residents. Part of the summer preparation is to augment its health personnel, oftentimes obtaining support from "retired" providers who have settled this island, which is reachable only by ferry or boat. While island residents love their waterways and see the increase of tourists as a welcome income source, health care providers view the summer months quite differently.

    a. How might health issues change with the different seasons and weather conditions on the island?

    b. Health services can also be obtained through the county hospital, which is located on the mainland. Explain how the weather and accessibility to the county hospital may impact health care access.

    c. What kind of benefits might be derived from water-related recreational activities, and what related health concerns associated with waterways?

    d. Given its location, hurricanes, nor'easters, and severe storms occur frequently. What weather-related issues might occur on the island? What health concerns might worry the year-round islanders?

REFERENCES—LOCATION

Cambridge Dictionary. (n.d.). Topography. https://dictionary.cambridge.org/us/dictionary/english/topography

Center on Society and Health, Virginia Commonwealth University. (2015). North Carolina 1 highway, 5 counties, 7 years of life [PDF]. https://societyhealth.vcu.edu/media/society-health/pdf/LE-Map-NCarolina.pdf

Office of Disease Prevention and Health Promotion. (2019). Access to health services. HealthyPeople.gov:https://www.healthypeople.gov/2020/topics-objectives/topic/Access-to-Health-Services

NC Budget and Management, Facts and Figures. (n.d.). Estimates of total population of North Carolina, North Carolina counties, and municipalities within counties for July 1, 2017 [Excel File]. https://files.nc.gov/ncosbm/demog/muniestbycounty_2017.html

Ricketts, III, T. C. (2002). *Geography and disparities in health care*. https://www.ncbi.nlm.nih.gov/books/NBK221045/

Statista. (2019). *Population density in North Carolina from 1960-2017*. Statista: The statistics portal: www.statista.com/statistics/304724/north-carolina-population-density/

Statista. (2019). *Population density of the United States*. Statista: The statistical portal: https://www.statista.com/statistics/183475/united-states-population-density/

Statisticalatlas. (2019). Population of North Carolina. https://statisticalatlas.com/state/North-Carolina/Population

United States Census Bureau. (March 2015). Understanding population density. https://www.census.gov/newsroom/blogs/random-samplings/2015/03/understanding-population-density.html

World Population Review. (2019). U.S. states density 2019. http://worldpopulationreview.com/states/state-densities/

Worldometers. (2019). U.S. population (Live). https://www.worldometers.info/world-population/us-population/

REFERENCES—ROADS

Caller Times. (2016). Are railroad crossing gates needed in rural areas? https://www.caller.com/story/news/local/2016/11/18/railroad-crossing-gates-needed-rural-areas/93970576/

Congressional Research Service. (2018). Rural highways. [pdf] https://crsreports.congress.gov/product/pdf/R/R45250/4

Dictionary of Military and Associated Terms. (2005). Secondary road. https://www.thefreedictionary.com/secondary+road

Driving Tips. (n.d.). Curves and winding roads require extra caution for any driver. http://www.drivingtips.org/curves.html

Forbes. (2020, July 2). Travel watch: COVID-19 is spreading along interstate highways, per new research. https://www.forbes.com/sites/suzannerowankelleher/2020/07/02/travel-watch-covid-19-is-spreading-along-interstate-highways-per-new-research/?sh=3b3ca6ca6f05

Henning-Smith, C., Kozhimannil, K. B. (2018). Rural–urban differences in risk factors for motor vehicle fatalities. *Health Equity, 2*(1), 260–263, DOI: 10.1089/heq.2018.0006

National Public Radio. (n.d.). Special series on the road to safety. https://www.npr.org/2009/11/29/120716625/the-deadliest-roads-are-rural

National Rural Health Association. (n.d.). EMS services in rural America: Challenges and opportunities. https://www.ruralhealthweb.org/NRHA/media/Emerge_NRHA/Advocacy/Policy%20documents/05-11-18-NRHA-Policy-EMS.pdf.

Samsara. (2019). Animal crossing: Preventing wildlife-vehicular collisions. https://www.samsara.com/blog/animal-crossing-preventing-wildlife-vehicle-collisions

Traffic Safety Facts 2017 Data. (2019). *Rural/urban comparison of traffic fatalities*. https://crashstats.nhtsa.dot.gov/Api/Public/ViewPublication/812741.

United States Department of Transportation Federal Highway Administration. (1990). *Technical advisory T 5040-29 paved shoulders*. https://www.fhwa.dot.gov/pavement/t504029.cfm

United States Department of Transportation Federal Highway Administration. (1993). *Roadway widths for low-traffic volume roads.* [Report] https://www.hsisinfo.org/pdf/94-023.htm

United States Department of Transportation Federal Highway Administration. (2018). Vegetation control for safety. https://safety.fhwa.dot.gov/local_rural/training/fhwasa07018/

REFERENCES—AIR

Arcury, T. A., Lu, C., Chen, H., & Quandt, S. (2014). Pesticides present in migrant farmworker housing in North Carolina. *American Journal of Industrial Medicine*, 312–322.

Donham, K. J., & Thelin, A. (2016). *Agricultural medicine: Occupational and environmental health for the health professions.* https://ebookcentral.proquest.com

Encyclopedia Britannica. (1998). Urban climate. https://www.britannica.com/science/urban-climate.

Hendryx, Michael, Fedorko, Evan, & Halverson, Joel. (2010). Pollution sources and mortality rates across rural-urban areas in the United States. *Journal of Rural Health*, 383–391. doi: 10.1111/j.1748-0361.2010.00305.x

Loftus, C., Yost, M., Sampson, P., Torres, E., Arias, G., Vasquez, V., Hartin, K., Armstrong, J., Tchong-French, M., Vedal, S., Bhatti, P., & Karr, C. (2015). Ambient ammonia exposures in an agricultural community and pediatric asthma morbidity. *Epidemiology 26*(6), 794–801. doi:10.2307/26511730

Mirabelli, Maria C., Wing, Steve, Marshall, Stephen W., & Wilcosky, Timothy C. (2006, April). Race, poverty, and potential exposure of middle-school students to air emissions from concentrated swine feeding operations. *Environmental Health Perspectives, 1*(14), 4.

Owens, K., Feldman, J., & Kepner, J. (2010). Wide range of diseases linked to pesticides. [pdf], *30*(2).. https://www.beyondpesticides.org/assets/media/documents/health/pid-database.pdf

Tinling, Melissa A., West, J. Jason, Cascio, Wayne E., Kilaru, Vasu, & Rappold, Ana G. (2016). Repeating cardiopulmonary health effects in rural North Carolina population during a second large peat wildfire. *Environmental Health, 15*(12). DOI 10.1186/s12940-016-0093-4.

United States Department of Agriculture. (n.d.). *Animal feeding operations.* https://www.nrcs.usda.gov/wps/portal/nrcs/main/national/plantsanimals/livestock/afo/

United States Department of Labor. (n.d.). Occupational Safety & Health Administration. Youth in agriculture. https://www.osha.gov/SLTC/youth/agriculture/organicdust

United States Environmental Protection Agency. (n.d.). Particulate matter pollution. https://www.epa.gov/pm-pollution/particulate-matter-pm-basics

REFERENCES—WATER

American Ground Water Education. (2018). Rural well or public water supply. https://agwt.org/content/rural-well-water-or-public-water-supply

Centers for Disease Control and Prevention. (2020). Importance of water quality testing. https://www.cdc.gov/healthywater/drinking/public/water_quality.html.

Centers for Disease Control and Prevention. (2014). Private ground water wells. https://www.cdc.gov/healthywater/drinking/private/wells/index.html

Centers for Disease Control and Prevention. (2015, July 2). Overview of water-related diseases and contaminants in private wells. https://www.cdc.gov/healthywater/drinking/private/wells/diseases.html

Centers for Disease Control and Prevention. (2019). North Carolina vector-borne diseases profile (2004–2016). https://www.cdc.gov/ncezid/dvbd/vital-signs/north-carolina.html

Earthworks. (n.d.). Acid mine drainage. https://earthworks.org/issues/acid_mine_drainage/

KidsHealth From Nemours. (2015, April 15). Fluoride and water. https://kidshealth.org/en/parents/fluoride-water.html?WT.ac=p-ra

National Ag Safety Database. (n.d.). Rural water safety. https://nasdonline.org/1858/d001799/rural-water-safety.html

Targett S., Geertsema C. (2014, June 21) Personal watercraft injuries. *Sports Injuries.* (1–7). https://link.springer.com/referenceworkentry/10.1007%2F978-3-642-36801-1_282-2. https://doi.org/10.1007/978-3-642-36801-1_282-2.

Theodore Roosevelt Conservation Partnership. (2017, November 9). Farm runoff and why it stinks for sportsmen and fish. [Blog]. http://www.trcp.org/2017/11/09/farm- runoff-and-why-sportsmen-should-care-about-this-sht/

United States Environmental Protection Agency. (n.d.). Drinking water requirements for states and public water systems. https://www.epa.gov/dwreginfo/information-about-public-water-systems

United States Global Change Research Program. (n.d.). Vector-borne diseases. https://health2016.globalchange.gov/vectorborne-diseases

World Health Organization. (2017, October 31). Vector-borne diseases. https://www.who.int/news-room/fact-sheets/detail/vector-borne-diseases

Yang, L., Nong, Q. Q., Li, C. L., Feng, Q. M., & Lo, S. K. (2007). Risk factors for childhood drowning in rural regions of a developing country: a case-control study. *Injury Prevention: Journal of the International Society for Child and Adolescent Injury Prevention, 13*(3), 178–182. https://doi.org/10.1136/ip.2006.013409

REFERENCES—WEATHER

Ag Safety and Health. (2021). Cold-related conditions and agriculture. https://ag-safety.extension.org/cold-related-conditions-and-agriculture/

Center for Climate and Energy Solutions (n.d.). Wildfires and climate change. https://www.c2es.org/content/wildfires-and-climate-change

Centers for Disease Control and Prevention. (2018, September 13). Flood water after a disaster or emergency. https://www.cdc.gov/disasters/floods/floodsafety.html

Centers for Disease Control and Prevention. (n.d.). Heat-related illness. https://www.cdc
.gov/pictureofamerica/pdfs/picture_of_america_heat-related_illness.pdf

Climate Central. (2018, February 28) More downpours: Increase in heaviest precipitation
events. https://medialibrary.climatecentral.org/resources/more-downpours-2018

Climate Central. (2018, May 16). New normals. https://medialibrary.climatecentral.org/
resources/new-normals-2018

Climate Central. (2019, April 11). Heavy rainfall trends across the U.S. [Interactive map, Greenville,
North Carolina]. https://www.climatecentral.org/gallery/graphics/heavy-rainfall-trends-us

Harrison, C., & Popke, J. (2011). "Because you got to have heat": The networked assemblage of
energy poverty in eastern North Carolina. *Annals of the Association of American Geographers*,
949–961.

Medical Press. (2019, March 1). Major flooding can bring skin infection dangers. https://med-
icalxpress.com/news/2019-03-major-skin-infection-dangers.html

National Capital Poison Center. (n.d.). Mold 101: Effects on human health. https://www
.poison.org/articles/2011-oct/mold-101-effects-on-human-health

National Park Service/USDA Forest Service. (n.d.). Fire terminology. https://www.fs.fed.us/
nwacfire/home/terminology.html

National Snow and Ice Data Center. (2020). Snow and climate. https://nsidc.org/cryosphere/
snow/climate.html

New York Times. (n.d.). How much hotter is your hometown than when you were born? https://
www.nytimes.com/interactive/2018/08/30/climate/how-much-hotter-is-your-hometown.
html

United States Energy Information Administration. (2017, April 6). U.S. House households' heating equipment choices are diverse. https://www.eia.gov/todayinenergy/detail.php?id=30672

Figure Credits

IMG 2.1: Copyright © 2019 Depositphotos/Celli67.

Fig. 2.1: Source: https://societyhealth.vcu.edu/media/society-health/pdf/LE-Map-NCarolina.pdf.

Fig. 2.2a: Source: https://www.carolana.com/NC/Counties/lenoir_county_nc.html.

Fig. 2.2b: Source: https://www.carolana.com/NC/Counties/hyde_county_nc.html.

Fig. 2.3: Source: https://www.carolana.com/NC/Counties/beaufort_county_nc.html.

Fig. 2.4a: Copyright © 2011 Depositphotos/elenathewise.

Fig. 2.4b: Copyright © 2012 Depositphotos/lakov.

Fig. 2.5: CDC, "Mosquito-borne and tickborne disease cases, 2004-2018," https://www.cdc.gov/
ncezid/dvbd/vital-signs/north-carolina.html, 2018.

Fig. 2.6: CDC, "Tick vector-borne disease cases," https://www.cdc.gov/ncezid/dvbd/vital-signs/
north-carolina.html, 2018.

Fig. 2.7: Source: https://medialibrary.climatecentral.org/resources/more-downpours-2018.

Chapter Three

The Economical Factor

Introduction

The second factor in the Rural Health Framework is the economical factor. There are five elements that comprise the economical factor: income indicators, employment types, job characteristics, health insurance, and health resources. We start the chapter with a review of the element Income Indicators as a way of anchoring us in describing income comparisons. This is followed by a review of Types of Employment—specifically **industries**, **firm size**, and **job characteristics**. We will note that based on types of employment, there are **job characteristics** that directly impact health outcomes. We bring forth farming as a primary employment sector of agriculture and explore how the **job characteristics** and major health concerns are associated with this type of employment. The last two elements to be discussed are Health Insurance and Health Resources. As we proceed through the chapter, we will use our running case, along with learning activities, to highlight the impact that these five elements have on rural populations and overall rural health.

Income Indicators as an Element of the Economical Factor

The income of an individual or a family unit impacts one's health and ability to access health care without regard for whether they live in a rural or an urban area. As a basic view of this issue, we can say that when income

Learning Outcomes

After reading about the economical factor, the learner will be able to

- Identify the five elements that make up the economical factor.
- Explain how each of the elements impacts the health status and/or health care access of people living in rural areas.
- Analyze and apply the economical factor and the elements comprising the economical factor in an assessment of their contribution to rural health outcomes.

Key Topics

Learning about the following key topics will support you in achieving the chapter outcomes:

- **Income Indicators:**
  median household income, average household income, and poverty-level income
- **Types of Employment Industries:**
  goods producing industries, service producing industries, agriculture, and self-employment (non-agriculture related)
- **Job Characteristics:**
  poor take-home pay, pay fluctuation, no health insurance, poor benefits, and strains on the body
- **Types of Insurance:**
  individual health insurance, employer-sponsored health insurance, and government- based insurance
- **Health Care Resources:**
  hospitals, health departments, federally qualified health centers, social agencies, and health care professionals

RUNNING CASE

The Cost of Care

Meet Jane, Jim, and Jessie. Each of them has diabetes and live in rural areas.

Jane Fisher (43 years old) is a full-time English professor at the local community college. She has been with the English department for 13 years and lives in the county seat for County A (population 95,000).

Jim Holden (age 67) is a retired New York city cab driver. He moved back to his hometown upon his retirement, 2 years ago. His hometown is small (population 900) and situated at the far eastern corner of the county, about 35 minutes from the county seat.

Jessie Parker (age 33) is a single mom with twin boys, age 7. She rents a booth at the local beauty salon in Town B, population 2,300, situated about 45 minutes from the county seat in the lower southern portion of the county. She has been a hair stylist for 5 years.

is low, people may not have enough money for preventative health care and prescription medications. The result of not seeking preventative health care is a delayed diagnosis and more progressed illness, such as later stages of cancer. Not purchasing needed medications results in deterioration of previously identified health issues, such as diabetes becoming uncontrolled. Consider that although good nutrition is essential for healthy outcomes, even food purchases are affected by one's income. Low-income households gravitate to food choices that feed the most family members and immediately satisfy hunger. This is typically cheap foods high in carbohydrates and calories.

Low-income families living in areas without safe spaces to recreate and exercise become at risk for obesity. Yet safe housing in safe neighborhoods is unaffordable for many low-income families. The house structure itself may be in need of repairs. It may have a leaky roof, faulty wiring, or mold and mildew growth, potentially causing respiratory problems, a house fire, or injury. So in this section we will look at how living in a rural area adds another level of complexity as we learn about income indicators.

In this section we will explore three income indicators and how income influences the health every day of people living in rural areas. The three economic indicators are **median household income**, **average household income**, and **poverty level**. Through these economic indicators we will compare differences between people living in rural areas and people living in urban areas. For a more complete examination, we will also discuss the insight gained by comparing these indicators county to county and county to state.

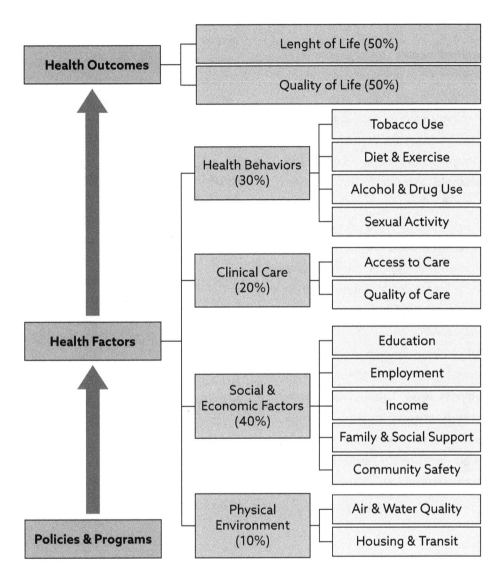

FIGURE 3.1   County Health Rankings Model.

REVIEW OF INCOME INDICATORS IN RURAL AREAS

Income data from 2015 showed people living in rural areas had lower **median household incomes** than urban households. The 2015 American Community Survey found that **median household income** in rural areas was $52,386, compared to urban areas at $54,296. The number of people making the **median household income** in rural areas was about 4% lower than the number of people in urban areas (American Community Survey, 2016).

Yet, people living in rural areas have a lower poverty rate (13.3%) than people living in urban areas (16%). Fewer people in rural areas live in poverty than people who live in urban areas (U.S. Census, 2016; American Community Survey, 2016). At a quick glance this data might

Median household income can be examined at the county level. It is the dollar amount on the income continuum where half of the households in the county earn more and the other half of the households in the county earn less. It is the midpoint on this income continuum. **Median household income** is not an average (County Health Rankings and Road Maps, 2019).

Average household income can be examined at the county level. It is all of the individual household incomes totaled together and then divided by the number of households in the county. It is a true average.

Poverty level can be examined at the county level. The federal government annually establishes the **poverty level**. The annual poverty level has two components: household income and number of people in the household. As an example, poverty level for 2021 could be stated as $26,500 for a family of four.

lead us to conclude rural poverty is less a concern. But in fact, when examining rural areas we must consider multiple economic indicators and to effectively plan health care resources consider the uniqueness of each rural community.

RELATIONSHIP OF INCOME INDICATORS AND HEALTH OUTCOMES

There is a relationship between income and health outcomes. Lower income is a predictor of poorer health outcomes. Examination of one income indicator does not provide a complete assessment. If we looked only at **poverty level,** we would be misled in regard to income in rural areas. While rural populations are poorer than urban populations, there are more people living at or below **poverty level** in urban areas than rural areas (U.S. Census, 2016). However, the overall rate of poverty is higher in rural areas than urban. By this we mean that given the number of people in a geographical area (e.g., a county), the percentage of people living in poverty in rural areas is higher

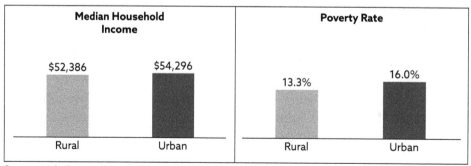

Source: U.S. Census Bureau, 2001-2015 American Community Survey.

FIGURE 3.2   Median Household Income and Poverty Level—Rural-to-Urban.

than the percentage of people living in an urban area (PBS, 2017). Thus, we must be very careful in how we describe poverty rates and in comparing poverty in rural and urban areas.

This highlights the point that several indicators require examination to understand the economic picture of a rural area. Then, for a better understanding of the area economy, collected county data should be compared with the same indicators for the state and region surrounding the county.

Section Review

As we leave this section, we note that people with incomes in the top half live 1.2 years longer than those with incomes in the lower half of incomes (Health Affairs, 2018). Low-income areas have less access to fresh foods, more fatty food restaurants, and fewer places to exercise (Health Affairs).

Our exploration of the economical factor continues with the element types of employment.

APPLICATION OPPORTUNITY

For designation of rural counties follow this link: https://www.ncruralcenter.org/about-us. Notice the North Carolina Rural Center provides three designations of counties based on population density. Let's compare the median household income in two counties, Tyrrell (rural) and Forsyth (urban). For county-level data about median household income, follow this link: https://data.ers.usda.gov/reports.aspx?ID=17828

What is the median household income for North Carolina?

What is the median household income for Tyrrell County?

What is the median household income for Forsyth County?

RUNNING CASE

Income Indicators

Jane Fisher: As a college professor, she earns $54,000 and is employed year-round with the community college. She lives with her husband, an accountant, and their 16-year-old son. The combined yearly household income is $104,000.

Jim Holden has a small monthly pension of $1,500 from his employment with the cab company. He also collects $1,700 monthly in social security income. He lives alone in a house he inherited from his dad.

Jessie Parker's income varies monthly. On good months, she earns $2,000 a month, but some months she earns as little as $400. Last year was not a good year for her, and she earned only $17,500. She receives no child support from the twins' dad, so her income is the only source of income for the family.

LEARNING ASSESSMENT—INCOME INDICATORS

Take this learning assessment and then compare your responses to the answers provided at the end of the book. You may find there are aspects of the element income indicators you would like to review to gain a better understanding.

1. List the five elements that make up the economical factor.
2. Consider the following statement: Ms. Jones is a 30-year-old, single mother whose income falls below the poverty level and who has no insurance. Select the answer providing data/facts distinguishing only the economical factor.
    a. 30 year-old, single mother, income below poverty level
    b. 30 year-old, single mother, without insurance
    c. Income falls below poverty level, female
    d. Income falls below poverty level, no insurance
3. The result of not seeking _____ health care is a delayed diagnosis and more _____ illness or disease process.
4. Select the response that best represents **median household income**.
    a. Median household income is the amount obtained by dividing the total aggregate income of a group by the number of units in that group. The means for households, families, and unrelated individuals are based on all households, families, and unrelated individuals, respectively. The means (averages) for people are based on people 15 years old and over with income.
    b. Median household income is the amount obtained by dividing the total aggregate income of a group by the number of units in that group. The means for households, families, and unrelated individuals are based on all households, families, and unrelated individuals, respectively. The means (averages) for people are based on people 21 years old and over with income.
    c. Median household income is the amount which divides the income distribution into two equal groups, half having incomes above the median, half having incomes below the median.
    d. Median household income is all of the individual household incomes for each of the households in the county totaled together and then divided by the number of households in the county. It is a true average.
5. **Poverty level** is set annually by the _____ _____ and is a stated as a dollar amount calculated based on the number of people in a household.
6. Explain how average household income is calculated for a county.
7. There are more people living at or below the poverty level in rural areas compared to people living in urban areas.
    a. True

    b. False
8. The relationship between income and health outcomes is proportional. Low income is associated with poorer health outcomes.
    a. True
    b. False
9. The economic picture of a county can be determined by simply looking at one of the three income indicators.
    a. True
    b. False
10. Name the three income indicators discussed in this section.

Types of Employment Industries as an Element of the Economical Factor

While in some areas the difference between rural and urban may be pronounced, overall the distribution of employment industries is similar between the two geographical units with the exception of farming. This section explores the types of employment industries found in rural areas, with special discussion of farming. Thus, the topics in this area include the types of employment and distribution of industries that employ rural residents; agricultural employment including jobs in farming, forestry, fishing, and hunting; and the role of small businesses and self-employment in rural areas. Health impacts associated with these employment industries will be discussed after this section, which will describe key **job characteristics** often associated with employment in these industries.

TYPE OF EMPLOYMENT INDUSTRIES

As with most things, there are differing opinions on how to classify the employment sector and occupational categories. For our purposes, we will use the United States Bureau of Labor Statistics' classification, which follows:

    a. Goods producing **industries**—wherein raw materials are transferred into goods. Within this classification are mining, construction, and manufacturing.
    b. Service producing **industries**—wherein personal and professional services are provided. Within this classification are retail, health care and social assistance, education, governmental jobs, leisure and hospitality, professional and business services, and wholesale trades to name a few.
    c. Agriculture to include farming, forestry, fishing, and hunting; both waged and **self-employed**. (Our focus will be a discussion of farming)
    d. Non-agriculture self-employment.

According to the Bureau of Labor Statistics, the vast majority of Americans (approximately 80% in 2019) are employed in the service-producing **industries**, followed by 14% in goods producing non-agriculture, then **self-employed** at about 5%, with agriculture-related **industries** accounting for approximately 1.2% of those employed (U.S. Bureau of Labor Statistics, 2020). Rural areas, similar to their urban counterparts, follow this distribution model with the exception that in many rural areas the agricultural **industries** employ a larger segment of the population.

There is no significant difference in the rural-to-urban distribution of **industries**. Instead, differences are noted in comparing rural-to-rural areas. While rural-to-urban differences may not be significant, often rural-to-rural areas are very different relative to the type of employment **industries** in their community. For instance, manufacturing may make up a larger employment proportion in rural areas closer to metropolitan areas while agriculture **industries** may account for a greater percentage of people employed in rural areas further from metro areas. Rural areas may also differ by region with agriculture found in middle America and the South and mining often having a greater employment segment west of the Mississippi River.

Some urban-to-rural differences emerge in employment **industries**. For instance, differences occur in the type and nature of small businesses. The classification of a business size (small business or larger enterprise) describes both the number of workers in the firm and the shared **job characteristics**. When we look at **firm size**, urban-to-rural differences are found. In rural areas, small businesses that often employ fewer than 10 employees may be opened more frequently by older owners (Fundera, 2018) or may represent a larger segment of immigrant owners. Differences also occur in self-employment. In rural areas, there are both actually less numbers and proportionally fewer people **self-employed** in the professional and business segment (e.g., accountants, health care providers, and lawyers) compared to urban areas (USDA Economic Research Service, 2020). Instead, it would seem that in rural areas there seem to be more rural residents that are **self-employed** in areas classified as personal services such as childcare, barbers/hair stylists, funeral directors, and landscapers to name just a few. Likewise, rural communities have a disproportionate number of discount retail

---

Industries: Classification based on the activity in which a firm/organization is primarily engaged. (We will rely on a four-industry classification system.)

Firm Size: Classification of a place of employment relative to number of employees (e.g., small business, large enterprise).

Self-Employed: Owns own business and thus works for self. May employ others or work alone.

Job Characteristics: Job features that manifest in and contribute to the nature of work.

stores (e.g., Walmart, Dollar General) as primary retail employers, which operate alongside small-business retail stores (e.g., independent grocery stores, antique shops, single-store clothing shops). Restaurants in rural areas tend to be smaller, fast-food, or fast-casual type eateries. While many rural restaurants provide excellent food, their settings may be smaller and their menu items less pricey.

According to the Small Business Administration, small business employs nearly half of all employed workers in the United States. While this fact is important everywhere, it is critical in rural areas that depend on small business to drive their economic engines. In general, small businesses in rural areas grow at a slower rate than those in urban areas. Rural small businesses may have small annual revenues, but have profits equal to or higher than urban small businesses (Fundera, 2018). Rural small businesses often face unique challenges in finding sufficiently well-educated workers, having readily available access to capital, and struggling with costs of employee benefits (e.g., health care) (Small Business Majority, 2010).

So we begin to see that rural areas depend heavily on small businesses. One reason is that rural communities have fewer large employers. For instance, rural areas rely on small-business retail, instead of many national chains (Daily Yonder, 2018). This reliance on small business has health implications, primarily through shared **job characteristics** that we shall review later in this chapter.

As an exemplar of employment in rural areas, let's explore farming as a sector of agriculture and a type of employment industry found almost exclusively in rural areas.

Farming is a source of rural jobs and influences the economy in rural areas. The United States Department of Agriculture (USDA) tells us there are approximately 2.05 million farming operations in the United States, with the average farm size about 444 acres. Between 2016 and 2019, these farming operations are collectively projected to generate $428 billion. So we see

> **Farming** is work performed by a farmer in conjunction with a farming operation.
> A **farm** is a place where at least $1,000 of agricultural products are produced and sold yearly.

that farms have an economic impact and obvious physical presence in rural areas. It will help us in the following section when discussing health issues related to **job characteristics** if we know the top farm commodities. These farm commodities determine the nature of the work and the physical environment of the work, which, in turn, predisposes farmers, farmworkers and farm families to certain health risks. In 2017, almost half (43.2%) of farm income in the United States came from growing corn and soybeans. Aside from crops, animal production also yields farm income. In 2017 cattle/calf produced the most income (38.3%), followed by poultry/egg (24.2%), and dairy (21.6%) (USDA ERS, 2019).

Farming as an employment sector in particular, has certain **job characteristics** associated with it as well as health issues that emerge from this type of employment. When we get to **job characteristics**, the nature of the farming tasks and commodities produced will be explained relative to health issues.

Section Review

So while the employment industries are similar in rural-to-urban comparisons, the companies, employers, and even the jobs themselves differ when comparing rural-to-rural. These differences will emerge as we discuss characteristics of jobs in the next section. One caution before leaving this section: occasionally when county data is reviewed, we find a list of major employers in the area. While such data is accurate, it is sometimes incomplete if our goal is to discover where rural residents are employed. For instance, when totaling the numbers, we notice that the number of employed residents does not equal 100% of all employed persons. Careful scrutiny reveals that nearly 30% of the workforce is missing. In our review, we notice that while names of major employers or employment industries are noted, small business and self-employment figures are absent. Although this may be understandable as the numbers represent major employers and do not represent small business or self-employment, it is important to carefully review employment numbers to ensure a full understanding of how residents earn a living.

A second caveat is the hint in this section of the impact that some employment industries may have on the community. For instance, if a larger employer in the community is education, then we can anticipate that the school will have a large social, fiscal, and political influence on the community. Similarly, the role of agriculture in a community may be disproportionate to the number of people actually employed in the industry. And we shall see in our upcoming discussion of the health resources, health care facilities have disproportionate economic influence in rural communities that goes well beyond employment figures. This is all to say that understanding the impact of employment industries in rural areas is more than accounting for major employers and the distribution of workers by industries (Daily Yonder, 2018).

LEARNING ASSESSMENT—TYPES OF EMPLOYMENT INDUSTRIES
Take this learning assessment and then compare your responses to the answers provided at the end of the book. You may find there are aspects pertaining to employment industries you would like to review to gain a better understanding.

1. Farming is a type of employment that is almost exclusively located in rural areas.
   a. True
   b. False

2. Agriculture as a broad type of employment includes which of the following: (Select all that apply.)
   a. Farming
   b. Fishing
   c. Forestry
   d. Hunting
3. List the four classifications of employment industries according to the United States Bureau of Labor Statistics.
4. Names two examples of self-employment in rural areas.
5. The types of self-employment in urban areas are the same as those in rural areas.
   a. True
   b. False
6. There is no difference in the rural-to-urban distribution of industries.
   a. True
   b. False
7. A farm is a place where at least _____ of agricultural products are produced and sold in a year.
8. Employment industries are similar rural-to-urban, but the companies, employers, and even the jobs themselves differ rural-to-rural.
9. Small businesses represent over 99% of employer firms and employ nearly _____ of all employed workers in the United States.
10. Explain why total data on a list of employers reported in percentages does not equal 100%.

Job Characteristics as an Element of the Economical Factor

As we have seen from the last section, many rural occupations fall within the service sector industry. Even for those that do not fall in this employment sector, rural jobs share similar characteristics and these characteristics have an effect on health outcomes. Here we will discuss the five **job characteristics** that most directly impact health outcomes: poor take-home pay, pay fluctuation, lack of health insurance offered by the job, few if any employee benefits, and strains on the body. These same **job characteristics** are shared by farmers, and we will utilize farming as an example to highlight how **job characteristics** relate to health concerns of farmers.

POOR TAKE-HOME PAY

The first **job characteristic** we wish to explore is the poor pay often associated with rural jobs. It is often said that rural jobs pay less and that rural workers make less money, sometimes a quarter of what urban counterparts make (Joint Economic Committee, 2018). At first glance, poor pay seems inevitable given the types of occupations and employers in rural areas—service industries jobs that traditionally pay less than other industries. Thus, it may not be surprising that many rural jobs pay at or below minimum wage, especially jobs like food service worker (waitress) or personal service worker (barber). These same jobs are low paying in urban areas, with the expectation that base salary is to be augmented through tips. While tips may significantly augment salaries of wait staff in metropolitan cities, tips are not usually large in rural areas and may not have the same income effect in rural areas as they do in more urban settings.

Another rationale often associated with poor-paying jobs in rural areas is the association between jobs and education. The narrative goes something like this: Rural residents have lower educational levels and thus qualify only for lower-paying jobs. Increase education, and salaries will go up. There is the unwritten expectation that increased education will close the gap between rural and urban pay. However, that is not necessarily the case. As can be seen in Figure 3.3, workers with the same educational level still earn less money in rural settings than similarly educated workers do in urban settings.

Although another often-cited explanation for this pay differential is the cost of living differences between the two settings, not all differences in rural-urban differences can be attributed solely to cost of living issues.

Instead, the more impactful issue is that rural jobs often cluster in more low-paying occupations and thus result in rural residents working in poorly paying jobs.

PAY FLUCTUATION

Not only are many jobs poorly paid, but rural employees are often subject to pay fluctuations (FAO). Sometimes called income variability or unstable income, rural workers often see large swings in their take-home pay over the course of the year. Why is that? One scenario is that workers may find themselves with differing take-home pay from week to week because the jobs themselves operate on a fluctuating schedule. For instance, a retail clerk may work a 29-hour shift one week, followed by a 15-hour shift the next week. Moreover, workers may not know how these hours will vary until the beginning of the work schedule cycle, sometimes only one week in advance.

Another type of pay fluctuation comes from seasonal variability in the job. Take for instance a realtor or landscaper who finds that some months there is very little work for them to do. While this is more predictable, the end result is that employee pay is unstable from month to month. This type of work differs from the formal category of seasonal employment where one knows more or less the exact time in which one is employed and time in which one is not employed (e.g., tour guide, school teacher). As can be expected, people who see pay fluctuations are more often the poor who are least able to tolerate inconsistent income.

Urban areas offered higher median wages for workers at all education levels in 2015

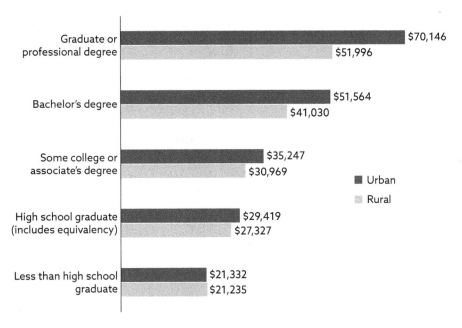

Note: Median earnings for all earners age 25 and older using metropolitan area definitions from the Office of Management and Budget.
Source: USDA, Economic Research Service using data from the U.S. Census Bureau's American Community Survey, 2015.

FIGURE 3.3   Urban Areas Offer Higher Earnings for Workers With More Education.

Pay fluctuation is important because income variability results in budgeting insecurities. Prescription medicines that were affordable when hours were higher or during peak work months may be reduced or eliminated as other household expenses become more immediate and critical—such as food and heating. Pay fluctuation also contributes to a lack of confidence around having sufficient funds to cover important but non-immediately critical expenses, such as private insurance. Lastly, pay fluctuation contributes to stress and the corresponding health outcomes associated with stress, both physical and emotional health concerns.

NO HEALTH INSURANCE
Rural jobs often do not provide employer-based health insurance. This may be due to the fact that employees do not work the required hours to qualify for health benefits or the fact that small businesses find paying for health coverage too expense. Regardless, the lack of health insurance coverage has a long-standing association with reduced health outcomes.

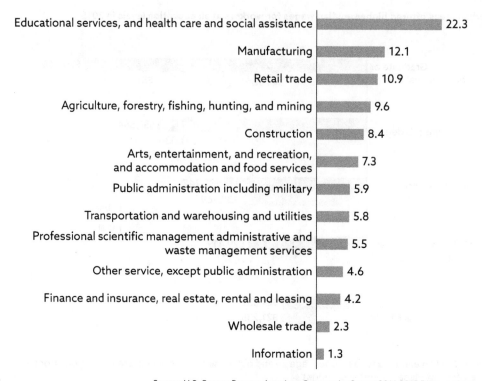

Educational services, and health care and social assistance   22.3
Manufacturing   12.1
Retail trade   10.9
Agriculture, forestry, fishing, hunting, and mining   9.6
Construction   8.4
Arts, entertainment, and recreation, and accommodation and food services   7.3
Public administration including military   5.9
Transportation and warehousing and utilities   5.8
Professional scientific management administrative and waste management services   5.5
Other service, except public administration   4.6
Finance and insurance, real estate, rental and leasing   4.2
Wholesale trade   2.3
Information   1.3

Source: U.S. Census Bureau, American Community Survey 2011-2015 5-Year estimates. For informaton on the ACS, see www.census.gov/programs-surveys/acs/

FIGURE 3.4   American Community Survey, 2011–2015.

A **seasonal job** employs workers during certain times in the year for a few weeks or months. Retail stores employ extra people during the Christmas shopping season to wrap gifts. In agriculture, jobs open up and employ workers to help only during weeks of harvest. These are temporary jobs with long work hours, unpredictability, and no benefits offered to the workers.

(See the later chapter on health insurance.) Health insurance plays a significant role in better management of chronic conditions, compliance with recommended screening protocols, and appropriate use of medical resources. Health insurance has been linked to longer life expectancy, greater positive health outlooks in self-reported surveys, and lower overall health costs. Cost impacted because without insurance, patients often present to emergency rooms (with its corresponding high health care costs) instead of seeing a primary care provider. Health is impacted because without insurance, patients often delay seeking care, making recovery more complicated. Thus, insurance is a prime factor in health outcomes for individuals. Yet, many rural employees work for employers that do not offer health insurance and have salaries too low to afford private insurance. So they go without.

POOR BENEFITS

Rural jobs provide fewer benefits. That is, rural employees do not have paid time off (vacation, sick, or personal time off), have fewer flex hours, have fewer supportive programs (e.g., employee assistance or referral programs), and have fewer opportunities to telecommute. While all benefits are important, we shall discuss two—paid sick leave and employee assistance programs—to illustrate the impact these have on overall health. Often associated with the type of work (e.g., food preparation or construction), lack of sick leave is linked to increased morbidity and overall decreased health status. If we stop to think about it, it makes sense. Without paid sick leave, employees must choose to lose a day's pay to go see a provider; they choose between ignoring pain and missing work for routine care. It is not surprising, then, that lack of sick leave is associated with decreased wellness visits (including immunizations), decreased utilization of preventive and screening care (e.g., mammography screening), and fewer follow-up visits—all associated with decreased health outcomes. Likewise, few rural employees have access to employee wellness programs that offer referrals for mental or addiction health care, which increase the likelihood of making lifestyle changes that reduce chronic illnesses and also increase employee productivity (ODPHP, 2017).

STRAINS ON THE BODY

Studies have shown that men who work in physically demanding jobs (e.g., construction workers) may suffer from premature deaths compared to those in sedentary jobs (Coenen et. al., 2018). We know that some jobs that require constant standing (e.g., retail clerk or hair stylist) or those that require constant repetitious movement (e.g., truck drivers, cashiers) aggravate arthritis and musculoskeletal disorders, such as wrist pain. Many jobs carry an increased potential for injuries from sharp objects, falls, burns, or inappropriate lifting of heavy objects.

APPLICATION OPPORTUNITY

One North Carolina study found as many as 40% of rural workers do not have access to paid sick days: https://www.policylink.org/sites/default/files/Employment_Equity_North-Carolina_06_19_18_0.pdf
Find rates for your area or state.

SPECIFIC JOB STRAINS FOR FARMERS

After having examined these five **job characteristics**, let's look at farming and how **job characteristics** specific to farming are related to health issues for farmers. If we ask a farmer to tell us about their most important farm asset and how they protect and take care of that asset, what would we hear? We would hear about the land and the quality of the soil and the time and effort they spend protecting the soil from erosion. Or perhaps we would hear an inventory of valued equipment and how they maintain and care for each piece. We would not hear a farmer describe themselves as the most important and valuable farm asset. However, the farmers and the farmworkers who work and live on the farms are the most important asset. Yet in day-to-day farming operations, preventative health care and safety are not typically placed first. Let's examine eight health issues experienced by farmers and consider how these **job characteristics** contribute to these health issues.

Depression

Research shows farmers and farmworkers have higher suicide rates than those in other occupations. The isolation of their jobs and the farming culture place them at high risk for anxiety, depression, and substance abuse. A 2017 study conducted by the American Farm Bureau Federation found 74% of farmers and farmworkers either personally or by knowing someone have been affected by opioid abuse, which is much higher than the overall adult rural population of 45% (Rural Health Information Hub, 2019). Feelings that outsiders do not understand the nature of farming add to the isolation. Fear of stigma prevents them from talking about their feelings. Farmers also experience generational pressure to keep the farm solvent and intact for current and future family generations. The success or failure of the farm has a ripple effect in families and in rural communities. Much lies outside the farmer's control. Commodity prices and the weather have a huge impact upon the farm's financial success, and farmers cannot control either.

Respiratory Issues

Farmers and farmworkers are at high risk for specific work-related lung problems, also referred to as occupational lung diseases. One common complaint amongst farmers is respiratory wheeze not caused by allergies. The changes in their respiratory tract are caused by inhaling fumes, dust, and chemicals that are present in their work environment. We know one in five farmers experience wheeze. Wheezing is a symptom that can indicate a continuum of respiratory problems. Two common agricultural work-related lung diseases are farmer's lung (or hypersensitivity pneumonitis) and idiopathic pulmonary fibrosis. Farmer's lung is caused by bacteria, molds, and fungi in hay and grain crops. Idiopathic pulmonary fibrosis occurs with repeated exposures to animal feed, dust, and agricultural chemicals. Progressive chronic respiratory disease can cause farmers and farmworkers to become disabled (Rural Health Information Hub, 2017).

Cancer

There are some types of cancers seen in farmers and farmworkers that have been shown to occur with exposures to specific agricultural crop chemicals. The cancers are lung, throat, thyroid, prostate, multiple myeloma, and non-Hodgkin's lymphoma. The workers that mix and apply chemicals to crops are most at risk for developing these cancers. We also know that the families have some level of health risk from exposure to the clothing of the chemical applicators. Lung cancer occurs, due to inhalation of diesel exhaust fumes. Farmers and farmworkers spend entire workdays operating tractors and other farm equipment and inhaling the diesel exhaust. In addition, farmers and farmworkers may develop skin cancer as a result of working in the sun. Lip cancer is seen, but cancers on the back of the neck are more prevalent (Agricultural Health Study, 2018).

Injuries

Farming is a dangerous industry. In 2017, there were 417 farmers and farmworkers who died out of the estimated 2,038,000 people employed full-time in agriculture (20.4 per 100,000) (CDC, 2020). We know that every day there are 100 nonfatal injuries that result in lost work time. A tractor rolling over on the operator is a leading cause of death. Deaths also occur from suffocation in grain bins and inhalation of poisonous gases in manure pits. Entanglement of limbs in machinery causes amputations. Less catastrophic injuries are slips, trips, and falls that result in sprains or broken bones. Workers fall from ladders, farm equipment, or grain bins. They trip over uneven terrain and surfaces when working in barnyards and fields. The interior surfaces of CAFOs are sometimes wet, causing falling. We know injuries occur more frequently among younger workers, those who work longer hours, those with hearing loss, or those who work with large livestock (Nat'l Ad Safety Database, n.d., Handling Farm Animals Safely). We should also recognize that farming is unique from many industries in that it can present health hazards to people not actively involved in the operation, such as family members living on the farm or visitors to the farm.

Hearing Loss

We already mentioned that hearing loss predisposes workers to injury, but we must also acknowledge that hearing loss is a common problem in farmers and farmworkers. They experience high decibel exposure from tractors, combines, and chainsaws. These noise sources can cause irreversible hearing loss over short exposure periods. Lower decibel exposures such as ATVs and animal noise can damage hearing over more prolonged periods of exposure (Nat'l Ag Safety Database, n.d. Hearing Loss).

Eye Problems

Eye problems are associated with working in CAFOs, cultivating fields, and applying chemicals. Farmers and farmworkers suffer from eye dryness and irritation from working in CAFOs and the resulting exposure to fumes and dust in these confined spaces. When planting or harvesting crops, dust and chemical residue are in the air, causing eye irritations. Farmers utilize agricultural chemicals to control weeds and insects. A typical method of chemical application is spraying. We know that age-related macular degeneration is associated with certain agricultural chemical that farmers apply to their crops (Donham & Thelin, 2006).

Exposure to Temperature Extremes

Long work hours spent outdoors places farmers and farmworkers at risk for health issues related to temperature extremes, both for heat and cold. In the summer months, the heat-related health issues are dehydration, heat exhaustion, and heat stroke. In the winter months the health issues become hyperthermia and frostbite. Heat-related illnesses are the most prevalent because planting season and the season of crop production occur in the spring and summer months (Donham & Thelin, 2006). Accomplishing the planting of crops and harvesting of crops is very time sensitive. When planting crops, farmers will work from the time the sun comes up until sunset and beyond.

Musculoskeletal Problems

Farmers and farmworkers overuse their joints, placing strain on muscles, tendons, ligaments, and joints. The nature of their work requires heavy lifting, pulling, bending, and squatting. They ignore pain and continue working, which results in joint deterioration and eventual arthritis (Donham & Thelin, 2006). Again, farmers place the work to be accomplished before their health. They work when in pain and injured. If it is planting season or harvest season, the work comes first and any pain or injuries are not treated.

These **job characteristics** also translate to barriers to health care for farmers and farmworkers. From an economic standpoint, farmers avoid seeking health care because a day away from work equates to a day without pay or potentially a loss of profits from crops. They may fear that missing a day of planting or harvesting will result in being fired. Without health care benefits, they are likely uninsured or underinsured, requiring the cost of the health care visit and treatment to be paid partially or totally out-of-pocket. For these same economic reasons, follow-up appointments are not typically feasible. Later we will explore the cultural factor and come back to farmers when discussing health beliefs and health values that can compound access to care.

Section Review

In the second element of economical factor, we reviewed type of employment (comprised by industry, **firm size**, and **job characteristics**) in rural areas. When thinking about rural health, it is critical to review where citizens are employed, the nature of that employment, and the **job characteristics** that impact health and health care access. Health care planning and interventions must attend to and anticipate these employment-related health issues in order to improve outcomes and access.

RUNNING CASE

Job Characteristics

Jane has both health benefits (insurance) as well as paid time off from her job. Thus, with sufficient notice, Jane can get coverage for her classes if she has to miss a class, or she can schedule her doctor's visits at a time she is not teaching. Her paid time off will help ensure that she can take advantage of referrals to nutrition counseling and to the diabetic educator.

Jim has a flexible schedule, so he should have a relatively easier time scheduling appointments—both with the health care providers and the diabetic educator or nutritionist. Jim's only limitation is not driving, so he will be dependent upon a friend or relative to take him to appointments. Last-minute cancellations may become a problem.

Jessie knows that she will have to block off available times on her calendar to schedule doctor's appointments or even referrals. As these appointments are often in clinics 45 minutes away, Jessie essentially has to block off an entire morning or afternoon, especially considering traffic on the road and delays at the clinics. While she intends to attend all appointments, calls from clients asking for special consideration often means that she will cancel her health care appointments in favor of good customer service and guaranteed income.

LEARNING ASSESSMENT—JOB CHARACTERISTICS

Take this learning assessment and then compare your responses to the answers provided at the end of the book. You may find there are aspects pertaining to job characteristics you would like to review to gain a better understanding.

1. List the five job characteristics that impact health outcomes.
2. In rural areas, the job characteristics predispose farmers to health issues. Select the answer that best describes the **job characteristics** and related health issue.
   a. Farmers and farmworkers experience respiratory illnesses.
   b. Farmers and farmworkers experience respiratory illnesses related to the inhalation of fumes from large equipment, confined animal feeding operations, and agricultural chemical fumes.
   c. Farmers and farmworkers have a high incidence of respiratory illnesses due to increased prevalence of cigarette smoking and vaping in this population.
   d. Farmers and farmworkers are more likely to smoke cigarettes and/or vape.

3. Farmers and farmworkers experience barriers to accessing health care. Name three job characteristics that make it more financially difficult for them to seek health care.

4. Workers with the same educational level earn less in rural settings compared to similarly educated workers in urban areas.
   a. True
   b. False

5. An impactful issue to understand is that _____ jobs often cluster in more low-paying occupations and thus result in rural residents working in more poorly paid jobs.

6. Name two examples of pay fluctuations.

7. Health insurance has been linked to longer life expectancy, greater positive health outlooks in self-reported surveys, and less overall health costs.
   a. True
   b. False

8. There were five examples provided to explain what is meant by **poor benefits**. List three of the examples of poor benefits.

9. Utilizing the three examples of poor benefits you provided in Question 8, explain how each impacts health status or health care access.

10. List five of the eight health issues of farmers.

Types of Insurance as an Element of the Economical Factor

Health insurance plays a significant role in better management of chronic conditions to compliance with recommended screening protocols to more appropriate use of medical resources. Health insurance has been linked to longer life expectancy, greater positive health outlooks in self-reported surveys, and less overall health costs (Common Wealth Fund, 2013). Cost is impacted because without insurance, patients often present to emergency rooms (with its corresponding high health care costs) instead of seeing a primary care provider. Health is impacted because without insurance, patients often delay seeking care, making recovery more complicated. Thus, it is critical to review the types and usage of health insurance in rural populations.

As we might expect, rural areas have patients with all sorts of health care insurance. In this section, we explore the types of insurance most prevalent in rural areas. To do so, we must first define the available types of insurance programs. Once we have done that, we can also describe the key impact that insurance has on health outcomes.

TYPES OF INSURANCE

At its broadest level, health insurance can be classified into three categories: insurance which we pay for ourselves (individual health insurance), employee-sponsored insurance (coverage that is available to employees through their jobs), and government-sponsored insurance (coverage made available to citizens through state and federal governments). The uninsured have an absence of insurance.

Private insurance is coverage provided by an insurance company and paid for by the individual, company or both. Within the private sector, there are two types of insurance coverage:

1. *Individual health insurance*. As the name implies, individual health insurance is health care coverage that is purchased and paid for by the individual. Persons are free to purchase their plans directly from a carrier (e.g., an insurance company like Blue Cross/ Blue Shield) or through a governmental exchange (HealthInsurance.org, n.d.).
2. *Employer-sponsored health insurance*. Employer-sponsored health insurance is coverage that is purchased by the employer and made available to employees. Both the employer and the employee share the cost of premiums associated with the offered plans, with the bulk of the payment made by the employer—as much as 80% for single coverage (People Keep, 2018).

In addition to private insurance, there is government-based insurance. Four major programs fall into this category: Medicare, Medicaid, military insurance (active and veteran), and Indian Health Services (Institute of Medicine, 2003). Here are general descriptions of these insurance programs.

1. *Medicare* is a federal insurance program which is primarily free for persons 65 and older and who have paid into the Social Security system for at least 10 years or have paid Medicare payroll taxes while working (established in 1965) (AARP, 2019). Persons with end-stage renal disease or other life-threatening diseases (e.g., Lou Gehrig's disease) may also qualify regardless of age.
2. *Medicaid* is an assistance program to help low-income children, pregnant women, and persons with disability, among others (Medicaid, n.d.). Qualification criteria are set by each state and vary nationally. Children's Health Insurance Program (CHIP) is another joint federal–state health insurance program for poor children through age 18.
3. *TRICARE* is a federally funded health insurance program for active duty military (and their families) and retirees under age 65 and their spouses or survivors (Medicaid).
4. *Indian Health Services* provides health services to members of American Indian and Alaskan Native tribes recognized by the federal government.

While these insurance programs are available in both rural and urban areas, the utilization of the programs varies.

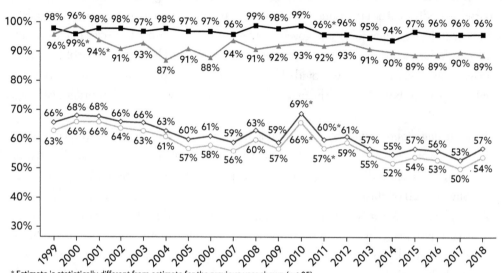

FIGURE 3.5   Percentage of Firms Offering Health Benefits, by Firm Size, 1999–2018.

PREVALENCE IN RURAL AREAS

While the vast majority of United States citizens are offered employer-based insurance (by some estimates as much as 80%), the distribution of who is offered employer-based insurance is dependent upon job type (Niskanen Center, 2019). That is, the percent of workers enrolled in employer-based health insurance increases with jobs in higher paying occupations.

In rural areas where there are a larger percentage of low-paying jobs, small businesses, or **self-employed** individuals, employer-sponsored private insurance is low. Instead, a larger number of persons with insurance rely on government-sponsored programs, especially Medicaid. By some estimates, nearly 24% of rural non-elderly persons were covered by Medicaid. That compares to 22% coverage in urban areas (Center on Budget and Policy Priorities, 2018). Those numbers are higher in poorer, more rural areas.

On the other hand, there does not seem to be a significant enrollment difference between Medicare beneficiaries in rural and urban areas. This may seem counterintuitive given that many rural areas have a disproportionate number of elders living in their region. One explanation may be that Medicare requires payment into the Society Security system, which may not occur for persons who are temporary or seasonal employees, **self-employed**, or have not worked outside the home and/or family-owned business. Similarly, rural TRICARE beneficiaries comprised only a third of all enrollees, although these enrollees tend to be more unemployed than their urban counterparts (Westat, 2018) and tend to have a harder time finding providers who will know and/or accept their insurance plan (Stars and Stripes, 2005).

Section Review

We know that health insurance is positively associated with better health outcomes. Persons with insurance are more likely to utilize preventive and screening services and to access these services more appropriately. Persons without insurance have worse outcomes for chronic illnesses such as diabetes or hypertension and die prematurely from specific diseases such as cancer. Without insurance, patients are less likely to access mental health services. Most problematic is a finding that uninsured persons face greater decrease in health status than those with insurance. (NCBI, 2002). Thus, the case is pretty clear: insurance is associated with health outcomes. So knowledge of insurance type and the impact of the prevailing type of insurance are critical when assessing rural health outcomes.

> **APPLICATION OPPORTUNITY**
>
> Using your county, calculate the number of persons enrolled in each of the type of insurance programs discussed here. Keep this information for use when comparing demographic information in later chapters.

RUNNING CASE

Types of Insurance

Faced with the diagnosis of diabetes, these individuals now know that they will be required to increase their health care clinic visits and prescriptions, as well as diabetes testing supplies. The type of insurance for these individuals has an impact on the cost of care for each person.

As an employee with the Community College, Jane has coverage with the school's Blue Cross/Blue Shield plan. She chose the 70/30 plan, thus has a copay of $40 to see her primary care physician and $95 to see her physician specialist for diabetes (endocrinologist). She has been ordered an insulin (Lispro), not covered by her insurance.

As an employee who paid into Social Security during the 20 years that he worked for the cab company, Jim has Medicare. Under Part B of Medicare, Jim pays $20 for doctor visits. He did not get a supplemental policy so he will have to pay out-of-pocket for all medications, including insulin.

Jessie does not have insurance. Her children are covered by Medicaid. When looking for insurance for herself, Jessie concluded that the individual plans were just too expensive, given her monthly fluctuating income. She knows that she will have to pay for all doctors' visits and medications herself.

LEARNING ASSESSMENT—TYPES OF INSURANCE

Take this learning assessment and then compare your responses to the answers provided at the end of the book. You may find there are aspects pertaining to insurance you would like to review to gain a better understanding.

1. Select the answer that best represents a person who would receive **Medicare**.
    a. A person who is 65 years old or older who has worked for a minimum of 10 years and paid into Social Security. A person may also qualify if disabled or diagnosed with end-stage renal disease.
    b. A person who is 65 years old or older who has worked for a minimum of 20 years and paid into Social Security. A person may also qualify if disabled or diagnosed with end-stage renal disease.
    c. A woman who is pregnant, the disabled, and children based on financial need.
    d. A young adult male whose earnings are below poverty level.
2. Select the example that represents a person who might qualify for **Medicaid**.
    a. A woman who is pregnant and has a 2-year-old child and is living in poverty.
    b. A young adult male whose earnings are below poverty level.
    c. A person who is 65 years old or older who has worked for a minimum of 10 years and paid into Social Security.
    d. A person who is 65 years old or older who has worked for a minimum of 10 years and paid into Social Security. A person may also qualify if disabled or has end-stage renal disease.
3. **Medicaid** is a type of government-based insurance.
    a. True
    b. False
4. Health insurance has been linked to _____ life expectancy, greater positive health outlooks in self-reported surveys, and _____ overall health costs.
5. List the three categories of health insurance discussed in this section.
6. What is the name of the federally funded health insurance program for active military?
7. There are more rural non-elderly persons who rely on Medicaid for health care coverage compared to their urban counterparts.
    a. True
    b. False
8. Provide an explanation for why there are not a greater number of rural elderly enrolled in Medicare compared with urban elderly.
9. Having health insurance does not impact health outcomes.
    a. True
    b. False

10. Thus, knowledge of insurance type and the prevailing type of insurance is critical when assessing rural health outcomes.
    a. True
    b. False

Health Resources as an Element of the Economical Factor

A major economical element is the presence of health resources: hospitals, health departments, **federally qualified health centers**, social agencies, and the like. In this section, we will look at one—**rural hospitals**—as illustrative of the economic impact of health care resources on a rural community.

HOSPITALS

In the United States there were approximately 6,090 hospitals in 2019. Of these, 514,142,621 were classified as a **community hospital** and 1,805 were classified as rural **community hospitals** (American Hospital Association, 2021). The economic impact of **rural hospitals** is significant.

- Often one of the leading employers in a rural area, **rural hospitals** provide well-paying jobs with benefits to local citizens. "On average, a Critical Access Hospital maintains a payroll of $6.8 million, employing 141 people. A 26–50 bed rural hospital employs 185 individuals and spends $11.8 million in wages, salaries and benefits on average, and hospitals holding 51–100 beds employ an average of 287 people and spend $19.9 million directly on those employees." (Rural Information Hub, 2020).

The presence of a hospital encourages corollary health businesses (e.g., pharmacy, home health services, expanded emergency personnel, medical supplies) to develop and flourish. In fact, by some estimation, for every job in the hospital, .5 jobs are generated in other businesses within the community. Moreover, hospitals may also encourage physicians to open outpatient clinics, further increasing the economic impact. It is reasonable to believe that a primary care physician may contribute as many as 23 jobs annually to the local workforce, generating over $1,500,000 in annual total revenue (salary, benefits, and purchases) (NCRHW, 2017). These are critically important jobs that cannot be replicated by other employers in the community.

Dollars generated directly and indirectly from a hospital provide tax revenues to improve schools and infrastructure, and drive economic development. These dollars raise home sales, boost retail revenues, and raise demands for local services and goods. A hospital signals the commitment of the community to a health workforce, thereby encouraging new business ventures to enter the area. In addition, increased health facilities reduce health costs for the patients. Workers have fewer hours lost from work and reduced costs to access health care

Community Hospital: **Community hospitals** include academic medical centers or other teaching hospitals if they are nonfederal short-term hospitals and accessible by the general public (American Hospital Association, 2019).

Rural Hospital: A **community hospital** located in a rural designated area (Athena Health, n.d.).

Critical Access Hospital: A subset of a rural **community hospital** that meets requirements by Medicare for CAH designation. Some requirements include the hospital providing emergency care 24-7; being at least a 35-mile drive from another hospital; and having fewer than 25 beds (Athena Health, n.d.).

Federally Qualified Health Center: A community based health center that provides primary care services to people in underserved areas on a sliding scale. A **Federally Qualified Health Center (FQHC)** may be a community health center, a migrant health center, a health care center for the homeless, or a health center for residents of public housing. The Health Resources and Services Administration funds these health centers and sets the requirements (HRSA, 2018).

(e.g., reduced transportation costs), and they often utilize health services more. In short, greater health facilities/resources not only improve health but directly contribute to the economic vitality of an area.

On the other hand, closure of **rural hospitals** or clinics has a devastating economic impact on a community. Unfortunately, **rural hospitals**, which often operate close to the margin, are great risk for closure. Difficulties recruiting or retaining health care providers, a patient mix overly reliant on federally funded health coverage plans (and the struggles that frequent policy changes ensue), increasing health care costs, and an increasingly medically complex patient population present challenges to **rural hospitals**. By some estimation, as many as 700 **rural hospitals** are at risk for closing, which would create what some call "medical deserts" (NRHA, 2016). While we have focused on hospitals in this review, similar economic impacts can occur from the establishment of other health care agencies: health departments, **FQHCs**, nursing homes). In later chapters, we will review strategies that may work to help maintain hospitals in an area.

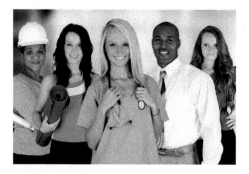

HEALTH PROFESSIONAL SHORTAGES

We cannot leave the health resources section without discussing health professional shortages. First, we must define the difference between health professional shortages in general and health professional shortage areas. The former is a lack of health professionals in an area regardless of discipline (e.g., medicine, nursing, pharmacy). The latter (HPSA) is a federal designation for shortages of primary care practitioners (medicine, physician assistants, and nurse practitioners) and dental and mental health providers. Designation of a HPSA area may carry benefits in terms of available grants or funding. For our template, we look at the bigger health professional shortage (with the expanded list of disciplines) to best represent the need of a rural community.

> **Health Professional Shortage**. A geographical area in which the ratio to provider is lower than what the discipline defines as optimal care/coverage.
>
> **Health Professional Shortage Area**. A geographic area, population, or facility with a shortage of primary care, dental, or mental health providers and services (HRSA, 2019).

Health shortages happen in all professions across urban–rural divisions. But, in rural areas, these shortages are acute. It is estimated that the physician–patient ratio is much higher in rural areas (NRHA). On average the physician to patient ratio is 271.6 per 100,000 people (Chiaravalloti, 2018), while in rural areas, the ratio may be as high as 1 physician to 2,500 patients (Becker's Hospital Review 2018).

This means more patients seen by each physician. Shortages also occur in dentistry where 60% of the dental professional shortages are in rural areas (Rural Health Information Hub, 2019). Similar numbers occur for a PA, NP, nurse, pharmacist, nutritionist, social worker, and the list goes on (Jackson, 2019). In later chapters, we will discuss how strategies such as expanding provider roles may help to close the shortage gap in rural areas.

Section Review

In reviewing health resources, it is important to note not just which health resources are found in a rural community, but the location of these resources. As mentioned in the geographical factor section, health resources may be concentrated in a county seat or a populace town, leaving citizens away from these centers with limited access. Thus, merely listing the resources is insufficient in determining the scope and benefit of health resources in a community.

Before leaving health resources, we should also note that while traditionally recognized health resources (hospitals, clinics, pharmacies) are important in rural areas, health resources may also take the form of community or social agencies. In many rural communities, there are Health Extension Regional Offices (HEROs) that are heavily involved in health education, worker safety programs, creation of health career pipelines, health care workforce development, grant writing, and in some cases assisting primary-care providers to reach community populations (Rural Health Information Hub, 2018; (Grumbach et. al. 2009). Community agencies (e.g., day care centers) and nonprofit organizations (centers for the visually impaired or Boys and Girls Clubs) as well as specialized social services programs (e.g., a school nurse, a lay health care worker, or a nurse in parish nursing) are also important health resources in the community. Collectively, these community services fill a void that is sometimes created by an absence of health care delivery resources such as a hospital, clinic or health department, especially in areas where resources are clustered away from some citizens.

RUNNING CASE

Health Resources

Jane is fortunate that an interprofessional team working with diabetic patients is part of the large multispecialty practice that is her medical home. Included on the team are several nutritionists, one of whom is a certified diabetic educator. When she schedules a visit, she can see several providers at the same time.

Jim's hometown has no health care providers per se. Instead, a mobile unit affiliated with the Academic Health Center comes from the neighboring county. Other than services provided by the mobile unit, residents must go to the county seat to get services. Fortunately for Jim, the mobile unit is equipped with telemedicine capabilities. If Jim wants to talk with a diabetic counselor or nutritionist or pharmacist, the nurse practitioner who staffs the unit sets the schedule for the telemedicine consults.

Jessie's community has a small family medicine practice affiliated with a larger FQHC located about 30 miles away. While the satellite clinic can follow her medical issues, other services like nutrition are only available at the FQHC. Unfortunately, the only certified diabetic educator is located at the county health center about 50 miles from where Jessie lives.

LEARNING ASSESSMENT—HEALTH RESOURCES

Take this learning assessment and then compare your responses to the answers provided at the end of the book. You may find there are aspects pertaining to health resources you would like to review to gain a better understanding.

1. Rural communities that have health care facilities realize economic benefits. Select the answer that represents an economic benefit.
   a. Increased utilization of alternative medicine
   b. Increased tax base
   c. Increased number of households with divorced couples
   d. Decreased distance to travel for health care

2. When a rural area gains health care resources—such as a clinic being established and health care professionals relocating there to live and work—there is an economic impact. (Select the best answer.)
   a. The tax base for the rural area increases.
   b. The access to care improves the health status of the people in the rural area.
   c. The rural area experiences a growth in new businesses and people moving to the area.
   d. All of the above.
3. Health professionals recruited to underserved rural areas may receive the following financial incentives to work in rural clinics and hospitals:
   a. Educational loan repayment from federal government.
   b. Higher cost of living in the rural area.
   c. Higher cost of houses and apartments.
   d. Higher paying job, as there is little competition.
4. Health professional shortages affect rural health by increasing travel expense, delaying care (thereby advancing disease stage), and increasing time needed to attend appointments (equating to more time away from work).
   a. True
   b. False
5. Shortages of health professionals in rural areas affect health status and/or health care access in the following ways: (Select the best answer.)
   a. Increase travel expense due to distance to receive care.
   b. More complex health care needs and advanced stages of illness due to delay in care.
   c. Increased time needed for appointments, resulting in more time off from work and missed wages.
   d. All of the above.
6. A primary care physician practice locating in area can contribute as many as 23 jobs annually to the local workforce, generating over $1,500,000 in annual total revenue (salary, benefits, and purchases).
   a. True
   b. False
7. Name two ways a rural community is impacted when their only hospital closes.
8. Explain the difference between a Health Professional Shortage Area (HPSA) and Health Professional Shortage (HPS).
9. How do the Health Extension Regional Offices (HEROs) serve as a health care resource in rural communities?
10. Name two community agencies found in rural communities that help fill the health care resource gaps.

CHAPTER SUMMARY

In this chapter we reviewed the five elements that comprise the economic factor: income indicators, types of employment (**industries**, **firm size**, self-employment, **and job characteristics**), types of health insurance, and health resources. To emphasize that the nature of employment type has health implications, we brought forth farming as a primary employment sector of agriculture exclusive to rural areas. We explored the job characteristics and major health concerns associated with farming.

We saw in our discussion how these elements intertwine. Jobs may pay poorly and carry no health insurance, thus forcing many rural families to rely on federal assistance programs like Medicaid or CHIPS. Further, we saw the positive impact that health resources have on an area, but also the toll that a financially impoverished area has on recruiting or retaining health professionals.

To aid in identifying all the economical elements, you are encouraged to thoroughly complete the Economic Factor Assessment Grid (see Table 3.1). Answering these grid questions not only allows you to fully describe the economics of an area, but also assists you when comparing one area to another. Likewise, activities at the end of the chapter and throughout the chapter are designed to assist you in applying the five economical factor elements to a rural area in your state.

Having discussed the economical factor and five elements also provides an opportunity to revisit the geographical factor in Chapter 2 and begin to build linkages between the two factors. Health resources located in some areas of the county may have a disproportionate burden to residents in other areas of the county. Employment that is clustered larger towns may require more residents outside the town to travel longer distances on rural roads. And of course, while income indicators are usually viewed in county data sets, great discrepancies may occur among towns within a county resulting in more pockets of disparities. The two factors are interwoven with each other.

As you complete the Economical Factor Assessment grid, you might want to use the same county that you used for the Geographical Factor Assessment Grid exercise. Doing so begins to paint a more comprehensive picture of your chosen location.

TABLE 3.1 Economical Factor County Assessment Grid Template.

Factor	Element	County Data	Source & Comments
Economical	Types of Employment	Major employers	
		Small businesses	
		Types of self-employment	
	Characteristics of Jobs	Hours	
		Benefits	

TABLE 3.1   Economical Factor County Assessment Grid Template *(continued)*

Factor	Element	County Data	Source & Comments
		Physical requirements	
		Health issues/risks	
		Full-time, part-time, seasonal	
	Types of Insurance	Veteran's Affairs	
		Private insurance	
		Employer insurance	
		Uninsured	
		Underinsured	
		Medicare	
		Medicaid	
	Economic Indicators	Average household income	
		Median household income	
		Poverty level	
		Total population	
		Net migration (increase or decrease in population).	
		Unemployed	
	Health Care Resources	Home care	
		Hospice, health department	
		Hospitals	
		Clinics	
		EMS	
		Fire/recue departments	
		Social services programs	

TABLE 3.1   Economical Factor County Assessment Grid Template *(contined)*

Factor	Element	County Data	Source & Comments
		Types of and ratio of health care professionals	
		Telehealth	
		Farm extension service	

Source: *The Journal of Rural Health*, "Rural-Urban Difference in Workplace Supports and Impacts for Employed Caregivers," https://doi.org/10.1111/jrh.12309. Copyright © 2019 by John Wiley & Sons, Inc.

CHAPTER ACTIVITIES—LEARNING CHALLENGE

Below are two learning challenges designed to help apply the economical factor's elements in a systematic review. The learning challenges can be completed individually or in small groups.

Learning Challenge 1: Look over the running case, identify how much of a burden (financial, inconvenience, emotional) it is for each of the three individuals described in the case. Take into account the issues we discussed in Chapter 1 (placement of health resources in the county seat and actual distance to these resources; conditions of rural roads and their effect on accessing care; and weather issues that might impede access).

Learning Challenge 2: Imagine the following individuals and describe how factors of income indicators, job characteristics, insurance type, and health resources would impact each one described below:

   a. A farmworker diagnosed with hypertension
   b. A local high school football coach diagnosed with high cholesterol
   c. A waitress at your favorite restaurant diagnosed with a torn knee that requires a partial knee replacement

CHAPTER ACTIVITY—PRACTICE VIGNETTES

Below are four practice vignettes. Read the scenarios, and answer the questions following each scenario. These practice vignettes may be completed individually or in small groups.

Vignette 1: Tenisha, a 35-year-old woman, met her husband shortly after graduating from Shaw University. They both were lucky to find jobs in Raleigh, where he worked as a manager for a large investment firm and she worked as an assistant director for an arts nonprofit. When the children came, Tenisha became a full-time mom. Now, following a messy bankruptcy and an even messier divorce, Tenisha has decided to move home to Port Deposit, Maryland to be near her parents, sister, and family friends. But she is worried. Even though Tenisha has a college degree in history, she is not sure about finding working to support herself and her two children, 10-year-old Wesley and 12-year-old Faith.

 a. Describe the prevalent jobs/employers in Port Deposit. Characteristically, what kind of salary and benefits do these kinds of jobs provide?
 b. Define median income, and identify the median income level for a household of three in Port Deposit. How is income distributed in the population: evenly or unevenly? Why is that?

Vignette 2: Silvia is about to finish her physician assistant studies. She is considering moving to a rural community and has begun exploring Marion, Ohio. To aid in her decision-making, she has drawn a 30-mile radius around Marion and is exploring the kind of health care practices/facilities that exist there, as well as the types of medical insurance prevalent in the area.

 a. What is the poverty level and income distribution in the county? How does this compare to state statistics?
 b. List the types of health resources prevalent within 30 miles of the area. Consider the poverty data and income distribution data, and explain whether these health care resources are adequate for the county.

Vignette 3: Kinston, North Carolina, is a rural community attracting many retirees from neighboring cities. Several health systems have initiated discussions with Lenoir Memorial Hospital in Kinston about a potential partnership. Critical to the discussions are the health resources of the area.

 a. Describe probable insurance types available in rural areas.
 b. List the health resources in the area.

Vignette 4: Juan is a 27-year-old, currently unemployed fisherman living in Wanchese, North Carolina. Even before his layoff, Juan was barely making a living wage with yearly income of $12,000, which has been supplemented by his wife's income of $7,000 as a part-time clerk. He just found out that he and his wife will be expecting their first child in 7 months. While he hopes to be back on his feet financially by then, he wants the best care for his unborn infant now. So he has begun his search for available prenatal care.

 a. What kind of health insurance might Juan's family qualify for? How might this change if his wife stops working?
 b. How does Juan's occupation as a fisherman affect his usage of a health care facility? Would this be different if Juan were an undocumented worker?

Vignette 5: Shandra is 68 years-old and lives in Elizabeth City, North Carolina, where she works waitressing during the day and cleaning offices part-time at night.

    a. Describe the potential type of health insurance that would be available to Shandra.

    b. Describe the job characteristics that pertain to the type of work Shandra does.

REFERENCES—INCOME INDICATORS

County Health Ranking & Road Maps. (2014). County health ranking model. https://www.countyhealthrankings.org/county-health-rankings-model

County Health Rankings & Road Maps. (2019). Median household income. https://www.countyhealthrankings.org/explore-health-rankings/measures-data-sources/county-health-rankings-model/health-factors/social-and-economic-factors/income/median-household-income

Health Affairs. (2018). Health, income, & poverty: Where we are & what could help. https://www.healthaffairs.org/do/10.1377/hpb20180817.901935/full/

Public Broadcasting Service News Hour. (2017). Six charts that illustrate the divide between rural and urban America.https://www.pbs.org/newshour/nation/six-charts-illustrate-divide-rural-urban-america

United States Census. (2016, December 16). Census Blogs: A comparison of rural and urban America: Household income and poverty [Census Blog]. https://www.census.gov/newsroom/blogs/random-samplings/2016/12/a_comparison_of_rura.html

U.S. Census Bureau. (2016, December 8).New Census data show differences between urban and rural populations. https://www.census.gov/newsroom/press-releases/2016/cb16-210.html

REFERENCES—TYPES OF EMPLOYMENT INDUSTRIES

Daily Yonder. (2018, February 20). Rural areas more likely to have independent grocers. https://www.dailyyonder.com/rural-areas-likely-independent-grocers/2018/02/20/23997/

Fundera. (2018, June 25). Rural small businesses earn better profits and more financing vs. city ones. https://www.fundera.com/blog/rural-vs-urban-business-financing/

Small Business Administration Office of Advocacy. (2012, September). Frequently asked questions. https://www.sba.gov/sites/default/files/FAQ_Sept_2012.pdf

Small Business Majority. (2010, February 12). Examining the unique opportunities and challenges facing rural small businesses. https://smallbusinessmajority.org/our-research/entrepreneurship-freelance-economy/examining-unique-opportunities-and-challenges-facing-rural-small-businesses

United States Bureau of Labor Statistics. (2020). Employment projections. https://www.bls.gov/emp/tables/employment-by-major-industry-sector.htm

United States Department of Agriculture Economic Research Service. (2019, November 27). Farming and farm income. https://www.ers.usda.gov/data-products/ag-and-food-statistics-charting-the-essentials/farming-and-farm-income/

United States Department of Agriculture Economic Research Service. (2020). Business and industry. https://www.ers.usda.gov/topics/rural-economy-population/business-industry/

REFERENCES—JOB CHARACTERISTICS

Agricultural Health Study. (2018). 2018 study update. https://aghealth.nih.gov/news/2018.html

Centers for Disease Control and Prevention. (2020). NIOSH—Agricultural safety. https://www.cdc.gov/niosh/topics/aginjury/default.html

Coenen P., Huysmans M. A., Holtermann A., et. al. (2018). Do highly physically active workers die early? A systematic review with meta-analysis of data from 193,696 participants. *British Journal of Sports Medicine 52*,1320–1326.

Donham, K. J., & Thelin, A. (2006). *Agricultural medicine occupational and environmental health for the health professions.* Blackwell Publishing.

Joint Economic Committee. (2018). Investing in rural America. https://www.jec.senate.gov/public/_cache/files/ed5bf0b5-dd14-473f-acdc-fd86ba98a6e1/investing-in-rural-america.pdf

National Ag Safety Database. (n.d.). Handling farm animals safely. https://nasdonline.org/44/d001612/handling-farm-animals-safely.html

National Ag Safety Database. (n.d.). They're your ears protect them—hearing loss caused by farm noise is preventable. https://nasdonline.org/1938/d001885/they-039-re-your-ears-protect-them-hearing.html

Office of Disease Prevention and Health Promotion. (2017, May 17). Five reasons employee wellness is worth the investment. https://health.gov/news/blog/2017/05/five-reasons-employee-wellness-is-worth-the-investment/

Rural Health Information Hub. (2017, August 23). Rural agricultural health and safety. https://www.ruralhealthinfo.org/topics/agricultural-health-and-safety

Rural Health Information Hub. (2017, October 4). Pulmonary health in rural America: Cause and impact of work-related lung diseases. https://www.ruralhealthinfo.org/rural-monitor/occupational-lung-diseases/

Rural Health Information Hub. (2019, Jan. 18). Healthcare access in rural communities. https://www.ruralhealthinfo.org/topics/healthcare-access

REFERENCES—TYPES OF INSURANCE

ARRP. (2019, September 25). Health Medicare resource center—do you qualify for Medicare?. https://www.aarp.org/health/medicare-insurance/info-04-2011/medicare-eligibility.html

Center on Budget and Policy Priorities. (2018, August 13). How Medicaid work requirements will harm rural residents—communities. https://www.cbpp.org/research/health/how-medicaid-work-requirements-will-harm-rural-residents-and-communities

Common Wealth Fund. (2013, June 21). The effects of health insurance on health: What we can expect from the Affordable Care Act. https://www.commonwealthfund.org/blog/2013/effects-health-insurance-health-what-we-can-expect-affordable-care-act

HealthInsurance.org. (n.d.). Glossary, "Individual health insurance." https://www.healthinsurance.org/glossary/individual-health-insurance/

Institute of Medicine. (2003). *Leadership by example: Coordinating government roles in improving health care quality.* The National Academies Press. https://doi.org/10.17226/10537

Medicaid—Keeping America Healthy. (n.d.). Medicaid. https://www.medicaid.gov/medicaid/index.html

NCBI. (2002). Institute of Medicine (US) Committee on the Consequences of Uninsurance. https://www.ncbi.nlm.nih.gov/books/NBK220636/

Niskanen Center. (2019, November 6). What's wrong with employer sponsored health insurance? https://www.niskanencenter.org/whats-wrong-with-employer-sponsored-health-insurance/

People Keep. (2018, November 8). What percent of health insurance is paid by employers?. https://www.peoplekeep.com/blog/what-percent-of-health-insurance-is-paid-by-employers

Stars and Stripes. (2005). Tricare struggling to find providers in rural areas. https://www.stripes.com/news/tricare-struggling-to-find-providers-in-rural-areas-1.36598Report2.pdf

Westat. (2018, April). 2017 Survey of veteran enrollee's health and use of health care. https://www.va.gov/HEALTHPOLICYPLANNING/SOE2017/VA_Enrollees_Report_Data_Findings_

REFERENCES—HEALTH CARE RESOURCES

American Hospital Association. (2021). Fast facts on U.S. Hospitals. https://www.aha.org/statistics/fast-facts-us-hospitals

Athena Health. (n.d.). What are community hospitals? https://www.athenahealth.com/knowledge-hub/community-hospitals/what-are-community-hospitals

Becker's Hospital Review. (2018, June 20). Fixing the medical staff shortage problem in rural areas. https://www.beckershospitalreview.com/population-health/fixing-the-medical-staff-shortage-problem-in-rural-areas.html

Chiaravalloti, Deborah. (2018, October 24). Physician shortages: Where they are & the most needed specialties. *Board Vitals.* [blog].https://www.boardvitals.com/blog/physician-shortages/

Grumbach, K., Mold, J.W.(2009) A health care cooperative extension service: transforming primary care and community health. *JAMA*. 2009;301(24):2589–2591. doi:10.1001/jama.2009.923

Health Resources & Services Administration. (2018, May). Federally qualified health centers. https://www.hrsa.gov/opa/eligibility-and-registration/health-centers/fqhc/index.html

Health Resources & Services Administration. (2019, August). Shortage designation scoring criteria. https://bhw.hrsa.gov/shortage-designation/hpsa-criteria

Jackson, Kate. (2019). The behavioral health care workforce shortage—sources and solutions. *Social Work Today*, 19(3), 16. https://www.socialworktoday.com/archive/MJ19p16.shtml

National Center for Rural Health Works. (2017). How economic impact supports health care. https://crh.arizona.edu/sites/default/files/u428/How_Economic_Impact_Supports_Health_Care_AZ_TUES_0.pdf

National Rural Health Association. (n.d.) About rural health care. https://www.ruralhealthweb.org/about-nrha/about-rural-health-care

National Rural Health Association. (2016, February 2). New report indicates 1 in 3 rural hospitals at risk. News release. https://www.ruralhealthweb.org/NRHA/media/Emerge_NRHA/PDFs/02-02-16PI16NRHAreleaseoniVantagestudy.pdf

Rural Health Information Hub. (2018). Health Extension Regional Offices (HEROs). https://www.ruralhealthinfo.org/project-examples/981

Rural Health Information Hub. (2019, March 22). Oral health in rural communities. https://www.ruralhealthinfo.org/topics/oral-health

Rural Information Hub. (2020, March 31). Rural hospitals. https://www.ruralhealthinfo.org/topics/hospitals

Figure Credits

IMG 3.1: Copyright © 2012 Depositphotos/rmarmion.

Fig. 3.1: Source: https://www.countyhealthrankings.org/county-health-rankings-model.

Fig. 3.2: US Census Bureau, "Median Household Income and Poverty Rate - Rural to Urban," https://www.census.gov/newsroom/blogs/random-samplings/2016/12/a_comparison_of_rura.html, 2016.

Fig. 3.3: USDA Economic Research Service, "Urban Areas Offer Higher Earnings for Workers With More Edication," https://www.ers.usda.gov/amber-waves/2017/july/urban-areas-offer-higher-earnings-for-workers-with-more-education/, 2017.

Fig. 3.4: US Census Bureau, "American Community Survey 2011-2015," https://www.census.gov/content/dam/Census/newsroom/blogs/2016/12/beyond-the-farm/fig01-type-industry.jpg, 2016.

Fig. 3.5: Niskanen Center, "Percentage of Firms Offering Health Benefits, by Firm Size, 1999-2018," https://www.niskanencenter.org/whats-wrong-with-employer-sponsored-health-insurance/. Copyright © 2019 by Niskanen Center.

Chapter Four

The Sociocultural Factor

Introduction

In this chapter, we will explore the third factor in the Rural Health Framework, which is the sociocultural factor. The five elements that make up the sociocultural factor include **beliefs and values, social capital, gathering places, faith-based organizations, and heritage and festivals**. In previous chapters we have explored elements that contribute directly to the health outcomes of rural residents, such as roads or income level, or elements where rural–urban differences impact differing health outcomes, such as job characteristics or marriages. Likewise, in this chapter, as we focus on the elements comprising the sociocultural factor we will include comparisons and relationships to health outcomes. While all five factors of the Rural Health Framework impact rural health, the sociocultural factor most influences the health care decision-making of rural residents. As we examine each of the five elements, we will discover that this factor tells us *who* rural people are and *what* they value and hold dear.

Additionally, we will explore initiatives that have been or can be used to partner in health planning to promote healthier lifestyles, promote disease prevention, or improve health services. This is a slight departure from previous chapters but provides for a better understanding of the sociocultural factor relative to health outcomes in rural areas. These five elements are distinctly important in rural settings and play a critical role in our understanding the health needs of people living in rural areas.

Learning Outcomes

After reading about the sociocultural factor, the learner will be able to

- Identify the five elements that make up the sociocultural factor.
- Explain how each of the elements impact the health status and/or health care access of people living in rural areas.
- Analyze and apply the sociocultural factor and the elements comprising the sociocultural factor in an assessment of their contribution to rural health outcomes

Key Topics

Learning about the following key topics will support you in achieving the chapter outcomes:

- **Beliefs and Values:**
  rural self-descriptors, description of health, alternative medicine
- **Social Capital:**
  family ties, civic engagement, religious affiliation, residents' intersection, informal leadership roles
- **Gathering Places:**
  barbershops and beauty salons, schools, volunteer organizations, local clubs, neighborhoods
- **Faith-Based Organizations:**
  trusted groups, grief support, gap services, partnerships
- **Festivals and Heritage:**
  community pride, local talents, fairs, health education

RUNNING CASE

4th of July Parade

Welcome to our annual 4th of July Parade. Before getting started, the Chamber of Commerce wanted me to remind everyone about the firework show tonight. Festivities kick off at 6 o'clock with a rousing rendition of patriotic songs by the Farmville Community Band. Bring the family out to hear the band. Hungry? No problem, Wally's Grill will once again be offering hot dogs and drinks. Oh, and the Scouts will once again be giving away fresh watermelon from 6 until they run out. So bring your lawn chairs and blankets and enjoy the music, the food, and the kid's activities sponsored by Parks & Rec. Yes, there will be face painting, balloon bounces, and sidewalk chalk drawings. And of course, the fireworks. Weather should be good, so we will start lighting up the sky at 9:15.

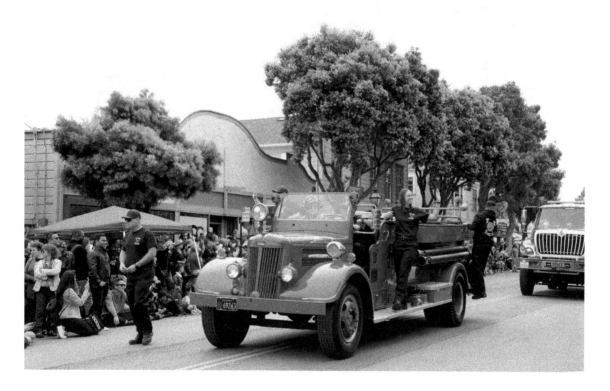

Prior to delving into the five elements associated with the sociocultural factor, let's explore what we mean when we speak of "**social**" and clarify how we are using the term "**culture**." The term "**social**" means those agencies or groups (e.g., community) that provide value to people or offer services/ resources needed or desired by people. **Social** settings provide a sense of the **culture** belonging to persons who are within those settings (for example, the parade pictured previously). For our discussion, we will rely on the classic definition of **culture**—the beliefs, actions, and patterns of behavior associated with a group of people. Moreover, we make the assumption that **culture** is not merely beliefs or feelings, but beliefs that drive actions—actions for the individual often reinforced by the group. **Culture** has an important role in the sociocultural factor as evidenced by relationships and the beliefs or values of rural people.

While distinct, **social** and **culture**, the concept that some settings promote a shared sense of values and behaviors underlie the main premise of the sociocultural factor. With this in mind, we will explore the elements that further define the sociocultural factor.

Social as applied to human society deals with the relationships of individuals or a group in society (*Merriam-Webster Dictionary*, 2020). **Culture** is the customary beliefs, social forms, and material traits of a racial, religious, or social group. **Culture** includes the characteristic aspects of everyday life shared by people in a place or a time period (*Merriam-Webster Dictionary*, 2020). **Sociocultural** means relating to or involving a combination of **social** and cultural factors (*Merriam-Webster Dictionary*, 2020).

Beliefs and Values as an Element of the Sociocultural Factor

RURAL SELF-DESCRIPTORS

The first element we will explore has to do with how a community and the people who reside in that community describe themselves and their way of life. As you remember, in Chapter 1 we asked you to list a series of words that you would use to describe "rural" and the people living in rural areas. Words that come to mind include people who know each other, who are family-oriented, who value **independence**, who are **self-reliant**, and who are **stoic**. In fact, these same descriptors that students used are used by rural residents to describe themselves. The top rural self-descriptors

---

Self-Reliance

The North Carolina coast is well known for its series of lighthouses that once guided ships traveling the Atlantic Ocean. Ship captains relied on these lighthouses for direction and landmarks to help avoid shipwrecks. Prior to electricity, the lighthouses were serviced by a lighthouse keeper and their family. Regardless of the weather conditions or the life circumstances, the keeper needed to fuel the light with oil and keep it burning. The job of the keeper was to overcome any and all obstacles to keep the light burning so that sea vessels could sail safely. Living remotely on islands, the lighthouse keeper and family had to provide all their own sustenance. They grew their own food, raised a few livestock, and served as teacher to their children and healer to anyone who got injured or sick. The lighthouse keeper and family lived on remote spits of land, isolated and cut off by water or impassible roads from neighbors. These keepers and their families epitomize the concept of **stoicism, self-reliance**, and **independence**.

Stoicism is defined as enduring pleasure or pain without showing emotion (Your Dictionary, 2018).

are independent-minded, self-sufficient, and stoic (Hillel, 2017). This is not hard to understand if we think back to earlier settlers of these small towns who had to rely on themselves for survival. A coastal lighthouse keeper is a perfect image to capture this sense of **self-reliance**.

While **values** of **stoicism**, self-reliance, and independence are noteworthy, these values do have a health impact, both good and bad. From the very best viewpoint, we might say these values are held by strong, hardy, capable people who can take care of themselves and those who rely on them.

But, we should also consider that persons who exemplify **stoicism** may ignore physical pain or mental illness. **Stoicism** can result in a delay in seeking medical care, therefore allowing the injury or disease process to worsen and more difficult to treat. A patient who is stoic can be difficult for health care providers to assess in terms of their level of pain or extent of their disease process. Mental illness may be viewed by a stoic person as concepts forbidden to be discussed or something to be hidden. Persons valuing **self-reliance** and **independence** exemplify optimism with can-do attitudes and honed problem-solving skills. Likewise, self-reliance and independence can also contribute to delays in seeking health care and a hesitancy to engage the help of health professionals.

The Latino people are a subculture prevalent in rural areas. While they are stoic and deny health care for themselves, they greatly prize the health and well-being of their children. They seek health care providers who demonstrate respect for them and their families. Latinos are more receptive to health care interventions when family members are included in the decision-making (Juckett, 2013). Now that we have expanded on how these values can impact the health status and health care access of people living in rural areas, let's explore the next issue, which is defining health.

DESCRIPTION OF HEALTH

If we ask you to define health, you might say something like "absence of diseases" or "feeling good." Your definition would be consistent with the Merriam-Webster definition of health

(*Merriam-Webster Dictionary*, 2020). A broader and more widely accepted view is that of the World Health Organization, which defines health as "a state of complete physical, mental and social well-being and not merely the absence of disease or infirmity." (WHO, n.d.). Both these definitions are frequently given by urban residents when they are asked to define health. Rural residents respond differently.

First, rural residents say that health is the ability to work hard and eat hardy. Therefore, by extension, rural residents consider being sick as meaning being unable to work and/or having loss of appetite. This view stems naturally from the descriptor of self-reliance and independence that we discussed above. One has to work hard and eat hardy in order to survive and to have a productive life (Coyne et al., 2006).

However, there are significant health implications from this belief. With this belief, rural residents' may not see the need for preventive care services; if one can work then no need to see a doctor (Coyne et al., 2006). As a corollary, if one is working and does not feel too sick to work, one may dismiss minor issues (pains, injuries, physical conditions) until they worsen. Likewise, one might dismiss silent illnesses (e.g., high blood pressure) for which there are few symptoms early in the disease progression. Both instances result in attending to illness much later in their disease progression, thereby increasing the likelihood of a more negative outcome from the illness/condition.

In addition to self-reliance and independence, rural residents describe themselves as being stoic. As a value, the idea is that one has to maintain a posture of positivism (everything will work out) and hide negative thoughts and feelings (worry, sadness). Hiding one's emotions and being tough are held in higher esteem than complaining or looking at the negative side of life. Unfortunately, **stoicism** may lead rural residents to overlook many health conditions, especially mental health conditions. Failure to express one's full range of emotions or to share concerns with another denies one the ability to seek help when it is needed, which is vital to achieving well-being and improving health (Coyne et al., 2006).

In addition to defining health as the ability to work, rural residents also define health as the ability to care for oneself and not be a burden to others. Rural residents want to be responsible for their own lives. While they might rely on others for an occasional emergency, not being a burden to family

---

Mental Health of Farmers

For instance, within the farming community there are higher rates of suicide than in the general population. One reason given may be the need to maintain a positive attitude when dealing with hardships (e.g., the weather, crop failures) that extend beyond the farming occupation to daily living. This stoic attitude may discourage realization of and discussion of issues like depression or suicidal ideation. Discussing mental health is taboo for farmers and never discussed outside the family (Hillel, 2017).

or the community is an important shared valued in many rural communities. They value their role in the family and consider fulfilling that role to be a demonstration of their well-being (Coyne et al., 2006).

ALTERNATIVE MEDICINE

Moreover, this idea of not being a burden may extend to health care providers; patients may not want to "burden the doctor" with minor issues. Many such patients prefer to administer home remedies to cure minor illnesses. While all emergencies should be immediately seen by a health care provider, we know that many rural residents still utilize more traditional home remedies. Therefore, it is important for a health care provider to ask patients what they have tried and to listen intentionally to their response. Many times, modern science has verified the scientific basis for these home remedies—for instance, chicken soup for a cold.

Other types of alternative medicine practiced by rural residents are chiropractic care, relaxation, meditation, herbal medicine, vitamins and minerals, and massage (Mundo et al., 2002). Rural people mistrust physicians, particularly if they are from another **culture**. People living in rural areas rely more heavily on family members and elders for health advice. To build trust, it is important for health providers to ask these patients about their home remedies and whenever possible include their alternative medicine therapies in the plan of care. This demonstrates respect for another person's **culture** and enhances the person's adherence to the plan of care.

Section Review

In this section we discussed beliefs and values as the first of the five elements comprising the sociocultural factor. We began with descriptive terms that rural residents used to describe themselves and gave the example of a lighthouse keeper. Next, we looked at ways that rural residents describe what it means to be healthy. Our exploration of the impact of beliefs and values ended with the role of alternative medicine therapies in rural populations.

LEARNING ASSESSMENT—BELIEFS AND VALUES

Take this learning assessment and then compare your responses to the answers provided at the end of the book. You may find there are elements of the sociocultural factor you would like to review to gain a better understanding.

1. List the five elements that make up the sociocultural factor.
2. Rural populations hold beliefs and values that influence their health care decisions and impact their health outcomes.
   a. True
   b. False
3. List three terms or self-descriptors that rural residents used to describe themselves.
4. Describe how stoicism can contribute to a rural resident's delay in seeking health care and how this might impact that individual health outcome.
5. Mental health issues such as depression and suicidal ideations are easily discussed among rural people.
   a. True
   b. False
6. When conducting a health history, health care providers should routinely ask rural patients about the use of home remedies and other forms of alternative medicine.
   a. True
   b. False
7. Identify four examples of alternative medicine therapies.
8. Select from the list provided a health belief or value held by Latino agricultural workers.
   a. Make annual visits to health care provider for wellness screenings.
   b. Believe in folk healers and utilize massage for pain relief.
   c. Find it easy to take medications prescribed by their health care provider.
   d. Commonly visit their health care provider when ill.

Social Capital as an Element of the Sociocultural Factor

The second element we will discuss is **social capital**. Life in rural areas is often seen as being higher in social capital. There is a greater sense of community and more social involvement. This social infrastructure is built upon the skills and resources of individuals living in rural areas. Social capital is best demonstrated when rural residents use these resources and skills to help others in need in the community in a reciprocal way. Mental health is improved when social capital is fully operational in a community. Consider the example of rural residents helping one another recover after a hurricane.

Example of Social Capital

Hurricane Dorian hit the coast of North Carolina in September of 2019, causing flooding in some areas and damaging tornados in others. Once Dorian passed through Carteret County, neighbors came out to help neighbors. They put their generators, chain saws, tarps, and tractors to work. Rural residents with generators to share powered up their neighbor's refrigerator and a few household lights. A local small-engine repair shop owner put the chain saws they had available in the hands of skilled rural residents that could work together and remove trees blocking driveways and yards. Anyone with a tractor came to provide horsepower for the debris removal. A neighbor with a several tarps helped a neighbor cover a hole in his roof. Churches organized meals for the community. Others got together and used their grills to cook food for neighbors and to share food supplies they had on hand.

While there are various definitions and perspectives relative to the concept of social capital, we will reply on the most foundational definition. Social capital is the relationship formed by persons that give meaning, strength, and resources to a person or group or community. This definition is in keeping with published work of contemporary authors on social capital (Social Capital Research, n.d.). But how are these relationships formed, and how does social capital provide a person with needed resources and reserves? The following analogy may help you understand more fully.

Think of social capital as a spider's web. Each thread of the web represents a relationship formed with family, friends, and peers at work. Likewise, relationships are formed between neighbors and friends as a result of membership in civic, religious, or professional organizations. Now, some relationships are stronger than others. For instance, most often, family relationships are stronger than more causal relationships such as those formed through membership on a soccer team. Returning to our analogy, the spider web with more and stronger threads provides a greater advantage in times of need.

In social capital terms, relationships in a person's life with breadth and depth provide similar safety nets in times of needs. In rural areas, where social and support resources may be scarce, the value of having a broad relationship network and one with depth affords resources otherwise not available: care assistance, financial help, child and family care, and transportation, to name just a few (Ziersch et al., 2009). Fortunately, evidence suggests that rural residents have and value strong social capital. Further, the research suggests several key venues to aid in the development of broad and strong relationships, some of which differ from those of their urban counterparts. Let's look at examples of key venues.

FAMILY TIES

It is logical that family members in closer proximity to one another have more opportunities to strengthen relationships and be available when needed. More than their urban counterparts, rural residents often have family members in closer proximity.

CIVIC ENGAGEMENT

Rural residents participate in civic engagement and feel more comfortable in their community. This may be because rural residents know their neighbors and feel safer in their communities.

RELIGIOUS AFFILIATION

Rural residents attend religious services more than their urban counterparts (Coyne et al., 2006). This allows rural residents to get to know one another and interact with others outside their family and neighborhoods. Faith-based organizations will be discussed more later in this chapter.

RESIDENTS' INTERSECTIONS

In smaller communities, rural residents have more opportunities to intersect as they engage in community life and fulfill responsibilities. A person might be involved in their child's PTO at school, serve as a scout leader or sport coach, be in the church choir or sit on a church board, join the chamber of commerce, or volunteer at the township fire station. The list goes on. But the reality is that smaller numbers of people in a community mean that there are insufficient people to fill all roles within the community without many citizens taking on multiple roles. While at times exhausting, overlapping membership allows the community to broaden resident relationships and strengthen relationships due to mutual interests/goals/activities.

INFORMAL LEADERSHIP ROLES

Each community has several residents who hold formal leadership roles within the community. The mayor or local pastors are two good examples of formal leaders. In addition, communities have informal leaders who help to broker information and effect change. Informal leadership roles include community voices and grapevine leaders. These informal leaders are respected and trusted to influence the opinions of those around them. Often the influence extends beyond changing someone's opinions to getting people to take some action. These informal leaders will speak up on an issue and through their stature and the respect that they engender help to set policy, direct resources, or achieve goals. In smaller communities where citizens know each other and have worked with many of the same people before, informal leaders are respected because they are known by the rural community rather than because of their position within an organization.

Community voices are people who are often sought out by researchers, key individuals in the community who have their finger on the pulse of the community. In many rural communities, business leaders, school personnel, faith-based organization members, and local political leaders seek out the individuals who serve as the voice of the community—those who simply always seem to know what is going on. Their insights, analysis, observations are critical. Many individuals known as community voices know what they know because of their continued involvement in the community.

Lastly, grapevine leaders are a type of informal leader in rural areas. A grapevine leader is plugged into these networks. They often know what is going to happen before it happens—or immediately thereafter. These informal leaders are indispensable to rallying support for candidates or a proposed action or helping to launch or curtail a plan. Intersecting memberships allow for these informal leaders to be known and, when appropriate, to be utilized to further the governance, growth, health, development, and safety of the community.

A word of caution about social capital: while it provides health benefits, it might also signal potential problems. Reliance on strong social capital might result in communities overlooking those that do not have such a resource: elders where family members and friends who have moved away, newcomers who have not had an opportunity to form such relationships, and those in changing family structures. We know subcultures such as immigrant Latinos may experience social isolation in rural communities. Latin American culture includes a strong sense of family and social ties. These relationships provide strong feelings of loyalty, cohesion, connection, and family as the center of life. The lack of these types of social capital, along with lack of rural infrastructure and resources, compounds the isolation of Latino immigrants in rural communities (Mora et al., 2014). There is evidence that social isolation has negative effects on health. Another subculture in rural communities might be single mothers without readily accessible childcare services. Single mothers often rely on family, friends, and neighbors for day care and after-school care. Thus, since social capital is important relative to health outcomes, when planning health care and allocating resources for rural areas, we must be sure to include various subcultures.

> **APPLICATION OPPORTUNITY**
>
> Create a social web of your relationships, and identify those threads that have the stronger impact. Explain how your web is strength and a caution.

Section Review

In this section we delved into social capital as the second element comprising the sociocultural factor. We learned that social capital can compensate for the lack of formal resources in rural areas and that there is health benefits to being socially connected. In contrast, we identified subcultures in rural populations that may be isolated and not benefitting from a social network. We noted that to avoid the negative health effects of social isolation, health planning in rural areas must include these subcultures in the community.

LEARNING ASSESSMENT—SOCIAL CAPITAL

Take this learning assessment and then compare your responses to the answers provided at the end of the book. You may find there are elements of the sociocultural factor you would like to review to gain a better understanding.

1. Rural residents have a greater sense of community and more social involvement than their urban counterparts.
   a. True
   b. False
2. Social infrastructure is built upon the _____ and _____ of individuals living in rural areas.
3. Social capital is the relationship formed by persons that give meaning, _____, and resources to a person or group or _____.
4. List key venues in rural areas that aid in the development of broad and strong relationships.
5. Give examples of formal leadership roles.
6. Community voices and grapevine leaders are examples of informal leadership roles. Explain how these informal leaders can be important to rural health.
7. Immigrant populations in rural areas may experience social isolation and are therefore at risk for being overlooked in allocation of health resources in rural areas.
   a. True
   b. False

Gathering Places as an Element of the Sociocultural Factor

Rural communities have several places within the community that afford citizens an opportunity to congregate, share information, influence viewpoints, and provide an informal but effective network of value sharing and information dissemination. In many communities, barbershops and beauty salons take on significant importance. Patrons feel safe in these spaces. There community members congregate and share important information. These places afford entertainment spaces as well. It is not unusual to see patrons engaged in card games or board games, patrons permitted to set up displays or demonstrations or patrons utilize the space for selling merchandise. Sometimes local leaders are invited to come in and talk with the patrons.

BARBERSHOPS AND BEAUTY SALONS

In Black communities, barbershops and hair salons have a unique and important role in the social life of the community. This knowledge of local customs coupled with the trust between barber and client makes the barber shop an ideal partner in health promotion. In one study, barbers were recruited to help promote prostrate education to their clients (Luque et al., 2015; Walden University Scholars Work, 2016). Likewise, Black cosmetologists have been found to be ideal partners in helping to educate their patrons on breast cancer and the value of early detection (Sadler et al., 2011). In rural communities, where there are limited resources for health education and health promotion, the role of gathering places like barbershops and beauty salons takes on an even greater importance (NMAAHC, n.d.).

SCHOOLS

Schools are another gathering place within rural communities. When discussing the demographical factor, we focused on the importance of community colleges in rural areas as sources of improving local educational levels. In this chapter about the sociocultural factor, we want to draw attention to the schools (high schools and community colleges) as avenues for social interactions in the community and potential health partners. In communities that have a high school, citizens gather to cheer local kids. There are Friday night football games, homecoming game night, school band performances, and PTO and other forms of parent–teacher associations. These events provide entrainment to the community, a sense of belonging, and a way to reconnect with friends and neighbors.

Gatherings such as these are important because they help to bind relationships and increase a sense of community. Because of the relatively small size of rural community populations, often citizens belong to various groups with overlapping membership. This is critically important for many health issues, such as disaster preparedness that relies on formal and informal channels of communication; relationship networks; and policies to ensure the best plans for the community.

VOLUNTEER ORGANIZATIONS

Volunteer organizations are found in many rural communities and help bridge the gap in resources to provide for the needs of their communities. Volunteer organizations, thus, play an important role in filling gaps such as fire departments and rescue squads. Volunteer fire departments and rescue squads provide the needed first responder services but also serve as integral as places to gather for community events. For example, rural people may gather at rural fire departments to raise money for families in need. Volunteer organizations draw rural residents together, who enjoy fellowship and donate to fundraising efforts through community barbecue plate sales and Brunswick stew sales.

LOCAL CLUBS

Rural areas have local clubs that build the character and skills of rural residents and serve as focal points for social gatherings. Local clubs may include the Ruritan Club dedicated to fellowship, goodwill, and community service. Homemaker Clubs bring rural women together to share or to learn food preserving, quilting, and managing the household. Youths can participate in 4-H clubs, taking on the responsibility of caring for and raising an animal to be later auctioned for money. Rural areas have livestock arenas where these young people can bring their calf, goat, or pig to be auctioned for school expenses. These events are well attended by many in the community, and bids are generous.

NEIGHBORHOODS

In addition to volunteer organizations and local club meetings, neighborhoods play a part as ready-made gathering places. Rural neighbors know each other better than urban neighbors, perhaps due to less population density compared to their urban counterpart and a greater degree of social capital. Rural neighborhoods are more homogeneous with many rural neighbors similar in terms of income level, education level, and even political beliefs (Pew Research Center, 2018). These neighborhood characteristics, while problematic on some level, also make neighborhoods a ready avenue for social interactions and communication sharing.

Section Review

In this section we discussed gathering places as the fourth of the five elements comprising the sociocultural factor. Communication building and relationship building take place where people gather. We began with the role of barber shops and beauty salons as places where patrons feel safe to share ideas and information. Also families frequent schools on regular bases. Other gathering places are volunteer organizations, local clubs, and neighborhoods. The gathering places frequented by rural residents become places to share health information and to learn about preventative health.

RUNNING CASE

4th of July Parade

But now back to the parade. Leading us off is the Mayor riding in a vintage police cruiser driven by our own Chief of Police. Here they come now. ...

Coming up next is troop 321 riding in the Piggly Wiggly Float. The troop just gets bigger and bigger every year. Just behind the float is a cavalcade of tiny cars driven by members of our local VFW. For you newcomers, the VFW has participated in every parade that I can remember—and I remember a lot of them. Just so you know, the Chief of Police has said that he will not be issuing any speeding tickets to the tiny cars—mainly because the cars don't go over 15 miles an hour. Immediately behind the tiny cars comes the high school marching band, cheerleading squad, and color guard. Let's give these youngsters a big round of applause for coming out to the parade even during their summer break and their parents who had to get up out of bed while on their summer vacation.

Oh, do I hear the fire truck siren! Just wait until to you see the truck—decked out in red, white, and blue steamers. The truck is flanked by marching first responders: volunteer firefighters, auxiliary EMS, and law enforcement representatives. If any of them get tired, the FWB Float right behind them has offered to give "a lift to all those that help us each and every day."

LEARNING ASSESSMENT—GATHERING PLACES

Take this learning assessment and then compare your responses to the answers provided at the end of the book. You may find there are elements of the sociocultural factor you would like to review to gain a better understanding.

1. Rural communities lack much of the formal types of public infrastructure found in urban communities.
   a. True
   b. False
2. Barbershops and hair salons are ideal places in rural communities to share health education topics. Explain why.
3. Schools in rural communities provide more than education. The events held at rural schools are entertainment places and build a sense of belonging.
   a. True
   b. False

4. Volunteer organizations in rural communities are gathering places but also fill service gaps like volunteer _____ department and volunteer _____ squads.
5. Give two examples of rural clubs that build character and skills of rural residents.

Faith-Based Organizations as an Element of the Sociocultural Factor

As has been mentioned, rural residents identify themselves as more religious. Rural residents attend religious services more than their urban counterparts (Coyne et al., 2016). Affiliation with a faith-based organization and participation in faith-based organization activities allow rural residents to know and interact with fellow residents outside their family, neighborhoods, or jobs. It is not surprising that within the Rural Health Framework, faith-based organizations are one of the five elements constituting the sociocultural factor. In some instances, although local citizens might not attend a church, synagogue, temple, or mosque, the mere presence of faith-based organizations adds an element of stability and community identity (Daman, 2018). Rural churches are often attended by multiple generations, becoming a means of transmitting and preserving community values and beliefs. Research proves that people of faith experience better health.

Historically, faith-based organizations played a significant role in the life of a small community. Just imagine the early beginnings of a small town. There was usually a series of homesteads scattered throughout the region with a central area located as the town. In the town, there was usually a general store, civic buildings (e.g., a courthouse and a jail, sometimes in the same structure), and of course, a church.

Churches—early faith-based organizations in small communities were most often churches or meeting houses—were a place where families could get away from the land and work. Families would make the trip into town to worship, to socialize with neighbors (think after service meet and greet, yearly homecoming lunches, special events like weddings and funerals, Sunday school and other educational events, and calendar events like Christmas). Attending church was perhaps one of the few social outlets available to rural families (Neitz, 2005).

Pastors and church leaders are well respected for the roles they play in the community: teacher, counselor, arbitrator, community leader, spokesperson, and advocate. Many civic and health organizations in a rural community (e.g., health boards) reach out to pastors for inclusion on the board for their input into important decisions and their influence. Their role and presence has been and continues to be critical.

PARTNERSHIPS

Thus, it is easy to understand that churches are places that encourage social interactions and that both the church and the leadership within the churches are some of the most trusted members of the community. Many churches embrace their role as partners in health by offering programs

Gap Services

- Assistance with transportation to medical appointments and health visits

- Emergency needs funds to help with heating, food, emergency travel, etc.

- Shut-in visitations and meal delivery

- Food banks

- Scholarship assistance for students pursuing college education

- Day care and elder care

- Pre-kindergarten education

and settings for health-related activities. In fact, churches have embraced the task of providing a variety of physical and mental health services for their congregations and the communities in which they are located. These activities include healthy cooking classes and health education programs. For instance, churches have been used to teach and promote evidence-based nutrition programs and to provide technical assistance to church members in implementing healthy lifestyle programs (Honeycutt et al., 2012). Churches have been used to implement diabetes and cardiovascular disease programs, especially some Black churches.

GRIEF SUPPORT GROUPS

Churches often sponsor support groups for many parishioners who have lost a spouse or a child. Led by a church member, these groups provide a form of bereavement ministry that addresses needs not met in the community where mental health professionals are scarce (Rawls, 2016). More specifically, churches might provide support groups for special populations, such as for families of persons with HIV/AIDS (Anderson & Shaw, 1994). Churches are ideal settings for these offerings, especially in communities where issues of privacy and anonymity might be problematic.

For instance, much research lacks participation of Black males, based on their historical mistrust of the medical system. In some instances, partnering with a church may help to recruit this valuable population so that better information and insights can inform later research (Carnahan et al., 2018). Conversely, churches may inform researchers on issues of importance that need investigation and funding. Rural churches have also undertaken what might be perceived as "gap services."

In many rural communities, the concepts of health and religion are heavily intertwined. Rural residents have indicated a preference for a holistic approach to health care, which includes addressing spiritual and religious health needs (Plunkett et al., 2016). Parish nurses might be among the best-placed registered nurses to capitalize on the existing strengths of rural churches and to promote the health of individuals in the communities in which they serve; they are well positioned to care for all dimensions of health, including both spiritual and mental health. Rural parish nurses are key community resources who can also help rural residents understand health issues and navigate the health care system (Plunkett et. al.).

In short, churches have a significant influence on the values and practice of the congregants and members of the church, as well as the community as a whole. They are available partners for health care programs. But when comparing rural faith-based organizations with urban counterparts, urban faith-based organizations are more likely to partner in health initiatives. With that being said, there seems to be untapped resources in rural communities. Special efforts need to be made to involve rural faith-based organizations more in health care initiatives and programs.

Section Review

In this section we discussed faith-based organizations as the fourth element making up the sociocultural factor. These organizations are important in rural areas because rural residents value religion and rely upon the religious community. Faith-based organizations offer grief support groups and fill gap services needed in rural areas. The gap services might be childcare, early childhood education, clothes, food, and emergency funds.

LEARNING ASSESSMENT—FAITH-BASED ORGANIZATIONS

Take this learning assessment and then compare your responses to the answers provided at the end of the book. You may find there are elements of the sociocultural factor you would like to review to gain a better understanding.

1. Rural residents identify themselves as being more _____ than their urban counter parts.
2. The presence of faith-based organizations in a rural community adds stability and community identity.
   a. True
   b. False
3. Research proves that people of _____ experience better health.
4. Pastors and church leaders are well respected for the role they play in rural communities. List four of these roles.
5. Churches provide a variety of physical and _____ health services for their congregations and communities.

Heritage and Festivals as an Element of the Sociocultural Factor

Many rural communities commemorate their history and cultural heritage through festivals. For instance, in North Carolina rural residents attend shad and shrimp festivals (in recognition of their coastal culture) (North Carolina Seafood Festival, 2020). A Meherrin Powwow and the state-wide Annual American Indian Heritage Celebration honors tribal people in the state. There are bluegrass dance and music festivals, a variety of watermelon and collards festivals (in recognition of the local harvest), and many dogwood festivals in recognition of North Carolina's state tree (Meherrin Nation, 2019). These festivals, small and large, bring together local residents, as well as citizens throughout the state, to help promote special cultural aspects of the community.

COMMUNITY PRIDE

Festivals are usually annual events that are anticipated and planned for throughout the calendar year. They create a time when bonds among public and private organizations, government, and neighborhood groups are forged and connections among elected officials, staff, volunteers and interested residents are generated. The community is engaged in building connectedness. Rural residents have emotional attachments to these festivals. Festivals evoke a positive feeling as people anticipate a fun family-oriented event. Rural festivals foster community pride and strengthen social capital types of relationships.

LOCAL TALENT

Festivals achieve other benefits. Festivals help local populations show off local talent, dancing, singing, craft-making, cooking, and athletic skills. Festivals help introduce festivalgoers to new ideas: tiny house communities, solar panels, new business ventures in the community, and changes brought about by climate change. Festivals have also become venues for health partnerships. Tables and booths that line the entrance to festival fairgrounds are perfect locations for distributing current health literature, which increases awareness about everything from safe water to immunizations to weight loss to action in case of a stroke (Hardy & Haithcox-Dennis, 2017). Tables and booths also provide a great community venue to announce new health and health care services.

In some communities, organizers create specially focused health care fairs. These events usually focus specifically on health-related activities and may include opportunities for attendees to receive health promotion information or get quick screen on a variety of health concerns such as cholesterol, blood pressure, and glucose. The fairs may help attendees connect with health care agencies and practitioners in their communities or learn about treatments such as opioid addiction programs. Health care fairs may be large events lasting an entire weekend or smaller afternoon events at local businesses or community locations such as the fire station.

FAIRS

Whether a county fair or state fair; no event better showcases rural heritage and culture of an area. Fairs have a variety of competitions—livestock, produce, flowers, and crafts are just a few—that reflect the lives and livelihoods of people in rural communities. A walk-through fairground building will find breeds of chickens that are raised in the region or prized swine, cattle, and mules. Fairs are usually held in the fall to recognize the completion of harvesttime and the beginning of a slower pace in farming communities as winter approaches. Crafts such as handmade furniture with caned seats and quilts with patterns passed down in families can be purchased or admired. Fairs are festive, with live music and firework displays that attract crowds for days.

HEALTH EDUCATION

In many agriculture-focused rural communities, county and state fairs are special. While providing fun activities, county and state fairs have a long history of including health-related activities. Cooking, baking, jam-making, and the like are often used not only to showcase cooking talents but to help educate entrants about safe cooking/preserving techniques and new food choices. Oftentimes, state agencies like Health and Human Services may have booths with focused health themes (e.g., Healthy Kids, Healthy Schools, Eat Less/Move More) that supply teachers and fair attendees with educational material, curricula, resource lists, and ideas for inclusion of health-related topics in the classroom. Sometimes there are demonstrations and staff development sessions that take place in these booths, equipping teachers and parents to go home with new information and a new skill set.

Section Review

We end our exploration of the sociocultural factor discovering how the heritage and festivals of a rural area reflect the people's culture and can impact their health status and health outcomes. Rural residents take pride in their heritage and their skills and talents passed down for generations. The festivals and fairs are anticipated all year and are viewed as fun family events. The rural events draw large crowds, creating for opportunity for health education and screening.

RUNNING CASE

4th of July Parade

No parade would be complete without live animals. The equestrian riders from Izzie's Stable are here to remind us how our town founders traveled long ago. Behind these wonderful animals come the clowns—some walking, some being pushed in giant strollers, and even one on a unicycle. And behind the clowns is the giant hay wagon with senior members of the 4th Club. The club wants to invite you all to come to the south side of the town square at the end of the parade for free hay wagon rides. They will be there as long as people want to ride.

LEARNING ASSESSMENT—HERITAGE AND FESTIVALS

Take this learning assessment and then compare your responses to the answers provided at the end of the book. You may find there are elements of the sociocultural factor you would like to review to gain a better understanding.

1. Many rural communities commemorate their history and cultural _____ through _____.

2. Festivals are a time when bonds among public and private organizations, government, and neighborhood groups are forged and where connections among elected officials, staff, volunteers, and interested residents are made.
   a. True
   b. b. False

3. List some types of current health literature distributed at booths located at entrances to fairs.

4. Fairs have a variety of _____ such as livestock, produce, flowers, and crafts that reflect the lives and livelihoods of the people in rural communities.

5. State agencies like Health and Human Services may have booths with focused health themes for teachers and fair attendees. List some of the resources teachers and fair attendees might find.

CHAPTER SUMMARY

In this chapter we reviewed the five elements that make up the sociocultural factor: beliefs and values, social capital, gathering places, faith-based organizations, and festivals and heritage. The culture and the heritage of a rural area can be overlooked when evaluating health needs. Somehow rural health research gravitates more to the hard data that economics and demographics yield. But we have seen in this chapter how important understanding rural people is to health planning. Each element and key concept explains how the sociocultural factor contributes to health concerns and health outcomes in rural populations. While these elements are significant independently of each other, most often the elements interconnect to form a more profound effect. Thus, it is important to comprehensively identify data for each of the elements in order to produce a complete picture of the rural community.

One way to ensure that we capture all the sociocultural elements is to complete the Sociocultural Factor Assessment Grid (see Figure 4.1). By answering each of the questions on the grid, no element is excluded or minimized; instead, the completed grid allows us to efficiently view key characteristics that are known to impact the health of the citizens of that county.

Not only can we use the grid to provide a snapshot of the sociocultural elements in the county, but we can use the grid to help us explain what we are viewing and even identify missing issues that might help inform us as to the nature of rural health needs. Tackle the two learner challenges at the end of this chapter to practice applying the Sociocultural Factor County Assessment Grid Template.

These factors and elements do not stand alone in their impact on rural health. In the next chapter we see how the demographical factor impacts health status and health care access of rural residents. In previous chapters we examined the impact of the geographical factor and the economical factor. Now, as we complete our understanding of the sociocultural factor on rural health, the journey of identifying issues that impact rural health continues in the next chapter.

TABLE 4.1   Sociocultural Factor County Assessment Grid Template.

Sociocultural

   Factor

	Health Beliefs and Values	Describe prevalence of: stoicism, independence, reliance on physical capabilities, relationships. Definition of health, use of home remedies, views of conventional health care.
	Social Capital	Identify and list social networks and support systems (formal and informal) found in the county.
	Gathering Places	Identify and list places where people gather in the county.
	Faith-Based Organizations	Identify and list any and all churches, mosques, temples, others. List some of the health-related initiatives these FBO present.
	Heritage and Festivals	Identify and list festivals held in the county. List any health-related initiatives that are part of these festivals. Find and summarize the information about the history and heritage of the area.

CHAPTER ACTIVITY—LEARNING CHALLENGE

Below are two learning challenges designed to help apply the sociocultural factor's elements in a systematic review. The learning challenge can be completed individually or in small groups.

Learning Challenge 1: Using your county or a selected county, complete the Sociocultural Factor Assessment Grid. Be sure to populate each element with comprehensive data elements. Data for the sociocultural factor will not be all in the form of numbers. The sources for facts/data about the county can be found at the county health department website and also at the chamber of commerce website. Be creative in your search by utilizing local newspapers. Look for the community calendar and local history for your county. Be sure to include all sources from which data/facts were obtained.

Learning Challenge 2: The Department of Health and Human Services has allocated funds to increase the immunization rates for your county. You have been asked to examine the sociocultural elements that might impact the decision-making of people in your county in regard to immunizations. Additionally, DHHS would like to know the best ways to access and make contact with local residents.

  a. Identify the elements pertaining to your county that would influence rural residents' decisions regarding immunizations. Explain why you chose these elements.
  b. Identify the elements pertaining to your county that would enhance the rural residents' accessibility to immunization programs.

CHAPTER ACTIVITY—PRACTICE VIGNETTES

Vignette 1: James and his family have worked on the Creswell's farm for 7 years. During the spring, they help in the cucumber fields, then they work in tobacco, and they finish the year with watermelons. At times, James has felt dizzy and light-headed, but he repeatedly refuses to go to the clinic to see a health care provider.

  a. Discuss how the personal beliefs within the farming community impact health care decisions.
  b. How might James define health, and what home remedies might James use prior to seeking medical care?
  c. Give examples of Washington County festivals and traditions that could provide opportunities for health screening and education.
  d. Discuss how James's health beliefs and values may delay him from seeking health care even when he is sick.

Vignette 2: Sally is a 52-year-old homemaker in Plymouth, NC. She volunteers often for her church and frequently prepares Sunday school lessons. She was diagnosed with type II diabetes 2 years ago.

a. Describe how rural culture may negatively impact Sally's ability to adhere to a diabetic diet.

b. Discuss how Sally's church may be utilized as a venue to positively impact healthy eating in the community.

c. In Washington County, what other events or places in the community where people gather could contribute to partnerships with the goal of healthy eating?

d. Discuss how Sally's health beliefs and values may impact her diabetes.

Vignette 3: Allen and Bonita are married with two children, Teresa, age 9, and Thomas, age 3. They have returned to the town of Everetts in Martin County to be near aging parents and continue the family farming operation.

a. What types of support systems would you expect to find in Everetts that might help Allen and Bonita with childcare during long workdays on the farm?

b. How might the concept of social capital in Martin County play a role in supporting or hindering Allen and Bonita's health outcomes.

c. Describe the common health beliefs of farmers that might facilitate or hinder accessing preventive health care.

d. Discuss how faith-based organizations in Martin County might function as a support network for this family.

REFERENCES—BELIEFS AND VALUES

Coyne, C.A., Demian-Popescu, C., Friend, D. (2006, October). Social and cultural factors influencing health in southern West Virginia: A qualitative study. *Prev Chronic Dis* [serial online]. http://www.cdc.gov/pcd/issues/2006/oct/06_0030.htm

Explore Integrative Medicine. (2014). An inside scoop on the science behind chicken soup and the common cold. https://exploreim.ucla.edu/wellness/an-inside-scoop-on-the-science-behind-chicken-soup-and-the-common-cold/

Hillel, R., Kraus, O., & Spencer-Thomas, S. (2017, October 4). Stoicism, stress, and suicide among farmers. https://www.sallyspencerthomas.com/dr-sally-speaks-blog/2017/10/3/stoicism-stress-and-suicide-among-farmers

Juckett, G. (2013). Caring for Latino patients. *American Family Physician, 87*(1), 48–54.

Merriam-Webster.com. (n.d.). Culture. https://www.merriam-webster.com/dictionary/culture

Merriam-Webster.com (n.d.). Health. https://www.merriam-webster.com/dictionary/health

Mundo, W. F., Shepherd, W. C., & Marose, T. D. (2002). Use of alternative medicine by patients in a rural family practice clinic. *Clinical Research and Methods, 34*(3), 206–212.

Your Dictionary. (2018). Stoicism. https://www.yourdictionary.com/stoicism

World Health Organization. (n.d.). What is the WHO definition of health? https://www.who
.int/about/who-we-are/frequently-asked-questions

REFERENCES—SOCIAL CAPITAL

Mora, D. C., Grywacz, J. G., Anderson, A. M., Chen, H., Arcury, T. A., Marin, A. J., &
Quandt,S.A. (2013, February 17). Social isolation among latino workers in rural north
carolina: exposure and health implications. *Journal of Immigrant and Minority Health, 16*,
822–830.

Sadler, Georgia Robins, Celine, M. Ko, Wu, Phillis, Alisangco, Jennifer, Castañeda, Shielda
F. & Colleen Kelly. (2011, August). A cluster randomized controlled trial to increase breast
cancer screening among African American women: the black cosmetologists promoting
health program. *Journal of National Medical Association, 103*(8), 735–45. doi: 10.1016/s0027-
9684(15)30413-2, https://pubmed.ncbi.nlm.nih.gov/22046851

Social Capital Research. (n.d.). Contemporary authors on social capital. https://www.social-
capitalresearch.com/literature/contemporary-authors/

Ziersch, A. M., Baum, F., Ngurah Darmawan, I. G., Kavanagh, A. M., & Bentley, R. J. (2009).
Social capital and health in rural and urban communities in South Australia. *Australian
and New Zealand Journal of Public Health, 33*(1).

REFERENCES—GATHERING PLACES

Luque, J. S., Roy, S., Tarasenko, Y. N., Ross, L., Johnson, J., & Gwede, C. K. (2015). Feasibility
study of engaging barbershops for prostate cancer education in rural african-american
communities. *J Cancer Educ., 30*(4), 623–628. doi:10.1007/s13187-014-0739-2

National Museum of African American History & Culture. (n.d.). The community roles of the barber shop and the beauty salon. https://nmaahc.si.edu/blog/
community-roles-barber-shop-and-beauty-salon

Pew Research Center. (2018). How urban, suburban and rural residents interact with their neighbors. https://www.pewresearch.org/social-trends/2018/05/22/
how-urban-suburban-and-rural-residents-interact-with-their-neighbors/

Sadler, G. R., Meyer, M. W., Ko, C. M., et al. (2004). Black cosmetologists promote diabetes
awareness and screening among African American women. *Diabetes Educ., 30*(4), 676–685.
doi:10.1177/014572170403000419

Walden University Scholars Work. (2016). Identifying the beliefs and barriers to
mammography in rural african women. https://pdfs.semanticscholar.org/151f/725f4776986e-
3a8b27b59e8a8a1357550904.pdf

REFERENCES—FAITH-BASED ORGANIZATIONS

Anderson, D., & Shaw, S. (1994). Starting a support group for families and partners of people with HIV/AIDS in a rural setting. *Social Work, 39*(1), 135–138. www.jstor.org/stable/23717034

Carnahan, L. R., Zimmermann, K., Manorama, M. K., et al. (2018, April). Physical activity and masculinity in rural men: a qualitative study of men recruited from churches, *Health Education Research, 33*(2), 145–154, https://doi.org/10.1093/her/cyy002

Daman, Glenn C. (2018, May 18). Why the rural church matters. https://factsandtrends .net/2018/05/18/why-the-rural-church-matters/

Honeycutt, S., Carvalho, M., Glanz, K., et al. (2012, September/October). Research to reality: A process evaluation of a mini-grants program to disseminate evidence-based nutrition programs to rural churches and worksites. *Journal of Public Health Management and Practice, 18*(5), p 431–439. doi: 10.1097/PHH.0b013e31822d4c69

Neitz, M. J. (2005). Reflections on religion and place: rural churches and american religion. *Journal for the Scientific Study of Religion, 44*(3), 243–247.

Plunkett, R., Leipert, B., & Olson, J. (2016). Exploring the influence of social determinants, social capital, and health expertise on health and the rural church. *Journal of Holistic Nursing, 34*(3), 236–243. https://doi.org/10.1177/0898010115605231

Rawls, Andrew S. (2016, May). Grief in community: The establishment of bereavement ministry teams from the congregation at Sandy Run Baptist Church in Mooresboro, North Carolina, *Divinity Projects, 28.* https://digitalcommons.gardner-webb.edu/divinity_etd/28

REFERENCES—HERITAGE AND FESTIVALS

Hardy, A., Haithcox-Dennis, M. (2017). Improving *Health Outcomes in a Rural Community. North Carolina Medical Journal, 78*(4), 258–261. doi: 10.18043/ncm.78.4.258

Meherrin Nation. (2019). Powwow & events. https://meherrinnation.org/13243.html

North Carolina Seafood Festival. (2020). Festival history. https://www.ncseafoodfestival .org/p/about/147

Figure Credit
IMG 4.1: Copyright © 2019 Depositphotos/Sheilaf2002.

Chapter Five

The Demographical Factor

Introduction

In this chapter we will explore the demographical factor. First we need to clarify the term "demographical" or "demographics," which has many meanings (e.g., descriptors or characteristics of a person and statistics about a population). In health research, demographics often include the five elements we will discuss in this chapter, as well as income level or residency. As these issues are discussed in other factors, this chapter describes the five demographical factor elements of age, race/ethnicity, gender, marital status, and education level. Each of these has a significant and proven impact on health outcomes and health delivery, substantiated through extensive research. It is not possible in this chapter to provide a comprehensive review of this literature, nor is that our intent. Instead, we want to concentrate on how these five elements manifest in rural areas and in so doing, highlight the rural health concerns associated with age, marital status, gender, race/ethnicity, and education level. We will also revisit many of the elements discussed in previous chapters to show the interconnectedness of the elements.

There are a lot of statistics in this chapter because of the nature of the five elements. To help us appreciate the human impact of these elements, each section will portray a rural citizen who manifests many of the issues presented in the element. The running case asks you to play the role of a panel member in a planning group charged with prioritizing health issues for your county.

Learning Outcomes

After reading about the demographical factor, the learner will be able to

- Identify the five elements that comprise the demographical factor.
- Explain how each element impacts the health status and/or health care access of people living in rural areas.
- Analyze and apply the demographical factor and the elements comprising the demographical factor in an assessment of their contribution to rural health outcomes.

Key Topics

Learning about the following key topics will support you in achieving the chapter outcomes:

- **Age:**
  children under 18 years and elders 65 years and older
- **Race/Ethnicity:**
  impact on health outcomes, racial/ethnical composition, health care barriers
- **Gender:**
  comparisons of overall health, health behaviors and health care access
- **Marital Status:**
  married, unmarried, cohabitation
- **Education Level:**
  impact on health care access, health outcomes, lifestyle choices

County Health Council Grant

The County Health Council meets to identify key county health concerns and potential resources to address these concerns. The Council comprises a representative from major health resources (e.g., a representative from the hospital and health department), two health providers, local opinion leaders (e.g., three pastors and a county commissioner), and four community members. Others attend as issues arise (e.g., a representative from law enforcement or the school system).

Council members have been notified that the next five meetings will be devoted to reviewing an announcement from the state Health and Human Services Division. DHHS is funding a series of pilot grants to address growing rural health concerns in the state. Each county will have an opportunity to apply for one of five rural health grants to address a key health concern in their county, based on county demographics and widely accepted health outcomes.

Read this running case and as you go through the chapter, think about where such a panel would get its information, what data you would want to review as a member of the panel, and how you would ultimately prioritize the five elements. We hope that by personalizing the data of these five elements we can visualize and better understand the people behind the numbers.

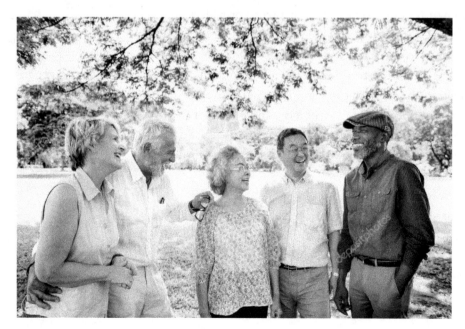

Age as an Element of the Demographical Factor

This section discusses **age** as one of the five elements comprising the demographical factor. The most prevalent age groups in rural areas are also two of our most vulnerable populations. Therefore key topics to be discussed in the coming paragraphs are **children under the age of 18 years** and **elders 65 years and older**. Let's begin with the element of age by looking at the people behind the numbers. Meet Jessie and Malcolm.

We will explore two **age distribution** groups or clusters: children under 18 years and elders 65 years and older. Each of these two age clusters represent unique challenges in rural areas.

Jessie is a 69-year-old retired postal worker who moved in with her daughter 2 years ago. While she has some health concerns (e.g., arthritis and COPD), Jessie is still able to care for her grandson, Malcolm, age 9, thus allowing her daughter to work rotating shifts at the local hospital. Jessie no longer drives, which at times is a bit confining as the family lives out of town on several acres of family land. As we go through this section, think about Jessie and Malcolm and how their health concerns might manifest themselves differently given their rural address than if they lived in the city.

CHILDREN UNDER 18 YEARS

Although in 2016, 13.4 million children lived in rural areas, this statistic is a bit misleading because so many more children in absolute numbers live in urban areas (USCB, 2016). Instead, review of age data at the county level often reveals children comprising a significant portion of the rural population, as much as a fourth of the total rural population. An interesting exercise is to pick rural counties at random and review **age distribution** within the counties. You may find results like those in these counties:

While not exactly a definition, there are several ways that age distribution is grouped: children under 5; children between 5 and 18; working adults 24–65; seniors/elders 65+. Be sure when you compare data that you are using the same groupings. For this chapter, we will classify children as persons under 18 years of age.

Herford County, North Carolina	25% of population under 18
Blanco County, Texas	24% of population under 18
Placer County, California	25% of population under 18
Sullivan County, New York	25% of population under 18

Thus, children become an important focus in rural health, especially as rural children and their urban counterparts are dissimilar in several significant ways. Rural children are less likely to receive preventive care and more likely to be overweight or obese. Rural children may receive less counseling on lifestyle issues (e.g., healthy eating, smoking, physical activity) (Georgetown University Health Policy Institute, 2017). Perhaps for this reason, more rural children smoke cigarettes than urban children.

Moreover, more than a fifth of rural children are poor, with roughly 25% of rural children reliant on Medicaid or CHIPS (Probst et al., 2018).This is important as children on public assistance, including Medicaid, often have greater difficulty obtaining health care referrals, perhaps due to health resources availability or cost of care. Some studies have suggested that poor, rural children have a higher incident of mental, behavioral, and developmental disorders than urban children (Probst, et al., 2018).

Rural children have higher mortality rates than urban children from non-homicidal unintentional injuries. It should be noted that while firearm injuries occur for both urban and rural children, urban children suffer more from firearm-related homicides than rural children. For rural children, unintentional injuries resulting in disabilities or deaths are often associated with motor vehicle accidents, farm equipment accidents (including use of heavy equipment or tractor rollover), or unsafe practices when driving ATVs or bicycles (Baernholdt et. al., 2012).

But things can go wrong, and there is rising frequency and poor outcomes associated with unintentional injuries for rural children. As we discussed in previous chapters, sustaining an accident in areas with longer wait times to EMS services certainly play a role in the intensity and outcome of

Here's a bit more about Malcolm, the boy we met earlier: Malcom is a good student with one passion: dirt bike riding. Every day after school, Malcolm jumps on his bike and rides around the property. The property is not big—a few areas of field and wooded areas with several low-lying areas where mud collects after rain. Malcolm likes to ride in the open fields; he sometimes ventures into the woods and down to the creek that borders his property and that of his best friend. Sometimes the two boys ride together, but most days Malcolm rides alone. His mother made him take a safety class offered by the local dirt bike group—but that was eons ago. And while Malcolm is careful, "Nobody can follow the rules ALL the time." Just using common sense is enough—after all, what could go wrong?

the injuries. Likewise, being in environments that might increase the possibility of an injury—such as walking on roads without walkways or shoulders and living in areas that support unsupervised ATV usage—may also contribute to this injury rate.

As mentioned at the onset of this chapter, there is a wealth of information about children's health and its subset, rural children's health. This is a very brief glimpse of the differences between rural and urban children's health with the intent of helping you appreciate that there are differences and that the differences may be understandable in light of the other elements previously discussed in this book.

> **APPLICATION OPPORTUNITY**
>
> Review elements from previous chapters discussing the geographical factor, the economical factor, and the cultural factor.
>
> Discuss which elements comprising the three factors would further impact either the health of rural children or the delivery of care to rural children.

ELDERS 65 YEARS AND OLDER

At the other end of the age spectrum are elders (persons 65 and older). As of 2019 data, 18% of rural residents are 65 or older compared to 15% in suburban areas and 13% in cities (Pew, 2018). While this clearly indicates that rural areas have large numbers of elders, some counties have a much higher proportion of their citizens in the elder category. This could be due to the fact that rural areas are popular retirement destinations with lower costs of living and a slower pace of life. Higher percentages of elders could also be due to improved overall health and the longer life span of current seniors. Lastly, many elder rural residents are not part of the emigration group that left rural areas for urban work environments, and as we noted in the previous chapters, rural residents are more inclined to remain in place, especially as they age. Regardless, rural areas have a growing elder population, and along with that population, the health concerns associated with geriatric care. Unfortunately, today's rural areas have insufficient social and health resources to attend to the needs of its elder populations.

Remember Jessie who moved in with her daughter? Once Jessie would have been surrounded by family members—aunts, uncles, grandparents, and cousins who lived near one another, sometimes sharing the same piece of family land. They would check in and care for older members. Moreover, many families had a relative who was available to move in with a needy family member. And if the family needed help, their "church family" was available. It was this culture of family caring for one another that reinforced the idea that elder members would best remain at home, cared for by family caregivers. There was not much cultural acceptance and little financial incentive to develop rural progressive-care retirement communities, nursing homes, or hospice centers.

However, Jessie lives in a very different world. She only has a few family members scattered throughout the community, and they, like her daughter, work full time. Nor can she count on her church family, as most members in the congregation are aging alongside Jessie. The reality facing Jessie is that geriatric services are scarce, public transportation is often nonexistent for rural residents who do not drive, and dual-income households and the out-migration of younger members of the family have resulted in fewer people available to provide assistance with daily living activities, medication checks, health care appointment transport, and overall family caregiving activities. This lack of family caregiving is particularly significant in an era of "age-in-place" literature touting both the desirability and benefit of non-institutional care.

> ### APPLICATION OPPORTUNITY
>
> Discuss how elements comprising the cultural factor contribute to or prevent worsening health effects for rural elders (see Chapter 4).

Not only are resources scare, but as elders age they also lose many social connections (e.g., church attendance, social community groups), thus reducing the positive effects of social capital (discussed in previous chapter) while increasing feelings of isolation that often lead to elder depression. It is no wonder that the CDC cautions that rural elders carry a high chronic care burden and face a greater chance of dying from preventable diseases due to their rural status (NC Health News, 2019).

Section Review

In this section we reviewed the element of **age** as the first of the five elements comprising the demographical factor. To turn numbers into people, we met Malcolm and Jessie as rural residents who are representative of the two **age distribution** groups: **children under 18 years** and **elders 65 years and older**. We explored the health concerns and health care access issues that children and elders face while living in rural areas compared to those living in urban areas. Through looking at data and facts about **age distribution**, we began our examination of the impact of demographics on rural health.

RUNNING CASE

County Health Council Grant

Meeting Agenda: Age-Related Services Grant

Council members read the following DHHS grant announcement:

The Age-Related Services Grant seeks to equip a rural community with focused health resources for one segment of their population (e.g., pediatrics, geriatrics, workman's compensation rehabilitation services). DHHS recognizes that as county demographics shift, community health resources may have gaps in services to specific age-related segments of the county. This grant will allow communities to develop new programs and services that focus on one segment of the county population.

Today's meeting focuses on reviewing the demographics of age distribution in the county, the identified health community.

LEARNING ASSESSMENT—AGE

Take this learning assessment and then compare your responses to the answers provided at the end of the book. You may find there are elements of the demographical factor you would like to review to gain a better understanding.

1. List the five elements make up the demographical factor.
2. Age distribution data can be grouped in several ways. Name the two age groupings that are discussed in this section.
3. When comparing data, as in age distribution, why would it be important to specify age distribution grouping of data?
4. Review of data at the county level often reveals children constituting as much as _____ of the rural population.
5. Urban children and rural children are dissimilar in significant ways. Select the responses below that accurately reflect these differences. (Select all that apply.)
   a. Rural children are less likely to receive preventative care.
   b. Rural children are more likely to be overweight.
   c. Rural children are less likely to receive counseling on lifestyle issues.
   d. Rural children are less likely to smoke cigarettes.
6. List the three sources of unintentional accidents that cause injuries resulting in disability or death in rural children.
7. Rural areas have a higher percentage of residents 65 years or older than urban areas.
   a. True
   b. False

8. List two examples of services or infrastructure that urban elderly have available to them that the rural elderly do not.

9. Rural elderly feel more isolated than urban elderly.
    a. True
    b. False

10. The CDC cautions that rural elders carry a high _____ _____ burden and face a greater chance of dying from _____ diseases due to their rural status.

Juan works as a cook and gladly cooks for family/friends. What he doesn't like is the restrictions that his diabetes and high cholesterol have put on what he can cook. Oh well, he is not alone. Seems like every week their Hispanic church is running another program on weight management or cooking without salt or carbs.

Ethnicity as an Element of the Demographical Factor

This section discusses **race/ethnicity** as one of the five elements constituting the demographical factor. To understand the importance of race/ethnicity relative to rural health, we will explore **health outcomes, race/ethnic composition, and health care barriers**. We begin this section by introducing Juan, who loves to cook.

HEALTH OUTCOMES

Do ethnicity and race matter relative to **health outcomes**? The answer is *yes*. Numerous studies have repeatedly shown a close association between race/ethnicity and health outcomes. For instance, studies have shown that racial/ethnical minorities self-report poorer health status and increased difficulty in seeing a provider due to costs. Rural minorities fare worse. Rural African American patients receive fewer cholesterol and cervical screenings than their urban counterparts, are more likely to be obese than urban residents, and are more likely to smoke (CDC, 2017). In fact, with the exception of binge drinking, racial/ethnical minorities report worse health in all categories than White, non-Hispanic respondents (HRSA, 2018_. We know that many of these health statistics are influenced by high rates of poverty among underrepresented populations. While there is some encouraging news that overall rural poverty rates have fallen for the past few years for all races and ethnicities, poverty rates among Hispanic and African American residents were higher in rural areas than in urban areas and higher compared to White, non-Hispanic residents.

We also know that poor health statistics are influenced by scarcity of resources, including shortages of health professionals. Health Professional Shortage Areas (HPSA), as we discussed in Chapter 1, is one way of measuring and comparing shortages across geographical areas. It is important to note that more than 80% of counties in which Hispanics or African Americans make up the majority population are designated as HPSA. The percentage is higher for Native American/Alaska Native majority counties (Probst et. al., 2004). This means that the lack of health providers coupled with higher poverty rates for Hispanic and African American citizens may serve to further reduce care for underrepresented communities. This may also help to explain the startling statistic that rural African Americans have higher mortality rates than urban African Americans and overall rural minorities have higher mortality than even rural Whites (non-Hispanic).

RACE/ETHNIC COMPOSITION

The race/ethnic composition of rural areas is changing. As of 2019, 20% of rural populations were racial/ethnic minorities. In fact, nearly 79% of rural residents were White, non-Hispanic, compared to 57% Whites, non-Hispanic, in urban areas (ERS-USDA, n.d.). This diversity picture, however, is not uniform throughout rural areas in the county (ERS-USDA, 2020).

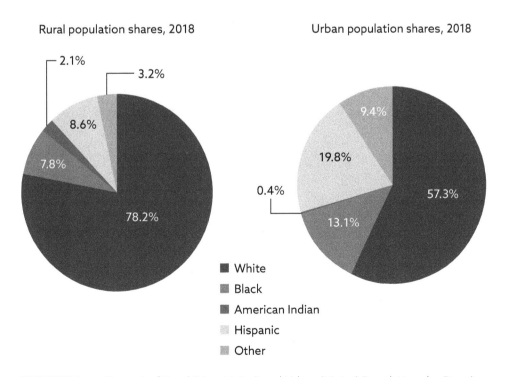

FIGURE 5.1   Percent of Rural (Non-Metro) and Urban (Metro) Populations by Race/Ethnicity, 2018.

In a border state like Arizona or Texas, Hispanics constitute the largest underrepresented group, while in Southern states like Mississippi, Alabama and North Carolina, African Americans are the majority of underrepresented populations (USDA-OMH). In fact, the United States Department of Agriculture predicts that while rural Whites and African Americans may be decreasing in number, rural Hispanic populations may be increasing (USDA, 2012). The 2020 Census will undoubtedly provide new figures reflecting the changing composition of rural citizens.

One word of caution when looking at race/ethnicity data: We must be cognizant that biracial births have increase substantially. Data collected in 2013 showed 7% of the population self-identified as biracial, with nearly half of that group under age 18. By some estimates, biracial identification is growing three times as fast as the population as a whole (Pew Research Center, 2015). We use the term *biracial identification* because unlike the historical classification in which biracial persons were expected to "claim" or be "designated" as one race, most biracial persons clearly view both races as equal and attribute "classification" to external factors (e.g., institutional bias) rather than self-perception. Rural areas may well see a significant rise in biracial populations, with the corresponding cultural and social changes that this may bring.

HEALTH CARE BARRIERS

Our discussion of race/ethnicity in rural health would not be complete without a conversation about trust. In addition to issues of resource scarcity, county composition, and income levels, health access is often a function of trust.

Data clearly shows underrepresented populations' historical mistrust of the health system: lack of confidence that one will be heard and understood, fears of historical abuse, and ongoing concerns about the level of care that providers give to those who are different (Musa et al, 2009; The Commonwealth Fund, 2021; The Hill, 2017). This mistrust (coupled with health beliefs from our last chapter about the cultural factor) serves as a strong deterrent from seeking care.

Let's return a moment to Juan. Juan's no-salt/low-fat cooking has gotten better. But he just doesn't feel well. Sometimes he gets a bit dizzy, and often he is really thirsty. His boss told him that he should see the doctor again, but Juan is hesitant. Dr. Richland is nice; not so nice is the mountain of paperwork that Juan must fill out each time he sees Dr. Richland—paperwork with questions that are hard to understand and sometimes hard to answer (e.g., address, phone number). More important than this paperwork is that Dr. Richland is always swamped—it's hard sometimes to get him to understand what Juan is trying to tell him. Take, for instance, the time that Juan was explaining how drinking boiled root water was good for his bronchitis. Dr. Richland just told him to take his antibiotics and leave the herbal stuff alone. Well. ... Juan doesn't feel all THAT bad. Maybe he just needs to carry a water bottle with him whenever he is away from home.

Rural citizens who are non-English speaking or come from different countries also have language barriers that make the health system incomprehensible and impede their comfort with seeking care. They may have culturally different views of when to seek care, when to use over the counter medications, and when to use home remedies. Some may fear legal repercussions for seeking care (e.g., may be undocumented).

> **APPLICATION OPPORTUNITY**
>
> Review the distribution of race and ethnicity data for your county. How does this distribution compare to state and national distribution data?

> **APPLICATION OPPORTUNITY**
>
> Think about Juan's reluctance to see a health care provider. What can be done to help increase Juan's comfort with and access to care?

Yet there is reason for concern among underrepresented populations. Hispanics have a 50% greater likelihood of dying from diabetes or liver disease than Whites, as well as 23% more obesity than Whites, and 28% less colorectal screening than Whites. While Hispanics smoke less and are less likely to have high blood pressure (if male), those who do have high blood pressure have it under less control (CDC Vital Signs, 2015). As many Hispanic patients reside in rural areas, these health statistics are of concern to rural health systems.

Section Review

In this section we looked at a second element of the demographical factor, the element **race/ethnicity** and its impact on rural health. Three key topics guided our exploration of race/ethnicity: **health outcomes, racial/ethical composition, and health care barriers**. Again we humanized the data by meeting Juan, helping us see a person predisposed to certain health outcomes while faced with health care barriers. We learned that the race/ethnic composition in rural areas is changing to reflect a growing Hispanic population. Likewise, data shows rural areas will see a rise in persons who identify as biracial. Understanding race/ethnicity data can help us anticipate the health needs of people who live in rural areas.

RUNNING CASE

County Health Council Grant

Meeting Agenda: Cancer Screening Grant

Council members reviewed the following grant announcement from DHHS:

According to the CDC, cancer rates are higher in rural areas, especially for colorectal and cervical cancers, both impacted by early detection and treatment. This grant seeks to implement pilot projects that increase the rate of screening for these two cancers, especially in ethnically diverse populations who traditionally do not get such screenings. Programs may address access to screenings, costs of screenings, distribution of screening resources, and education about the value of screening to underserved populations.

Today's meeting focuses on reviewing the demographics of the racial/ethnic distribution in the county, the increased rate of colorectal and cervical cancer within each racial/ethnic group, and model programs used elsewhere to encourage greater cancer screening participation.

LEARNING ASSESSMENT—RACE/ETHNICITY

Take this learning assessment and then compare your responses to the answers provided at the end of the book. You may find there are elements of the demographical factor you would like to review to gain a better understanding.

1. There is a close association between race/ethnicity and _____ _____.
2. When comparing health outcomes and health behaviors of rural African Americans to urban African Americans, which of the following are accurate? (Select all that apply.)
   a. Rural African Americans receive less cholesterol screening than urban African Americans.
   b. Rural African Americans receive less cervical cancer screening than urban African Americans.
   c. Rural African Americans are more likely to be obese than urban African Americans.
   d. Rural African Americans are more likely to smoke than urban African Americans.
3. The overall rural poverty rates have fallen in the past few years.
   a. True
   b. False

4. More than 80% of counties in which _____ or _____ _____ are the majority are designated as HPSA.

5. Rural African Americans have lower mortality outcomes than urban Blacks, and overall rural minorities have lower mortality outcomes than even rural Whites, non-Hispanics.
   a. True
   b. False

6. The United States Department of Agriculture predicts that while rural Whites and African Americans may be decreasing, rural Hispanic populations may be increasing.
   a. True
   b. False

7. By some estimates, _____ identification is growing three times as fast as the population as a whole.

8. List three of the barriers to seeking health care that underrepresented populations experience.

9. Hispanics have a _____% greater likelihood of dying from diabetes than Whites.

10. Compiling data and facts regarding the racial/ethnical populations in a county is important to understanding the health care needs.
    a. True
    b. False

Gender as an Element of the Demographical Factor

In this section we explore **gender** as one of the five elements that makes up the demographical factor. Three key topics will guide our exploration of gender and its impact on rural health: comparisons of **overall health, health behaviors, and health care access.** Through data we will see how rural women and men differ from their urban counterparts. As in previous sections, we will meet the people behind the numbers. Let's meet Mary, who is pregnant (see box on this page).

Approximately 35 million females (women and girls) live in rural areas. In terms of **overall health**, studies have shown that

Mary Ellis is excited about her pregnancy, but with her track record of miscarriages, she is also worried. This has heightened her ongoing anxiety disorder and really made sleep difficult. It has been weeks since she has slept the whole night. Once before when she had trouble sleeping, Dr. Patterson prescribed a sleep medicine that she could take as she needed it. Should she take some now even while pregnant? Better not. What should she do; whom can she ask? She hates to take time off from work, but being tired all the time is not good for her or the baby. She will just have to make the effort and endure the 45-minute car ride to Clifton to get a solid answer to her question.

APPLICATION OPPORTUNITY

Consider one health issue, such as intimate partner violence among rural women, and brainstorm geographical, economical, and cultural/social issues that might help explain this data.

rural women report poorer health status, report higher unintentional injuries, including higher rates of motor vehicle related deaths than urban women. Rural women have higher cardiovascular disease related deaths and higher incidences of cervical cancers. This may be due to the fact that rural women receive fewer of the recommended breast and cervical cancer screenings. As a result of this, rural women are more likely to have breast cancers diagnosed at a later stage. Like others in rural areas, rural women have higher rates of obesity than their urban counterparts (Committee Opinion No. 586, 2014).

Health care access impacts the health of rural populations. Shortages in rural areas negatively impact rural women's health, particularly the shortages of OB-GYN practitioners. Closures of rural hospitals also put pregnant women at greater risks, as they have longer distances to drive for care (e.g., almost half of pregnant rural women live within 30 minutes of a hospital offering prenatal care) and distance to hospital may encourage planned deliveries to avoid being caught in long commutes. Shortages of mental health providers may account for the fact that rural women face more frequent and more destructive intimate partner violence (Committee Opinion No. 586, 2014).

Rural residents in general are more likely to suffer from strokes, and rural women are at a greater risk for less favorable outcomes from strokes than rural men (Medical News Today, 2021). Women, in general, suffer more from depression than men, and rural women are especially vulnerable. Greater stroke **education** and awareness programs would serve both rural women and men. Rural women also have greater occurrences of intimate partner violence, either because of a greater culture of nondisclosure, fewer resources, less **education**, or a greater number of unhealthy lifestyle behaviors (e.g., alcohol consumption) (Peek-Asa et al., 2011).

In a comparison of men and women's health, women in general live longer than men—as much as 5 years longer. Current longevity ages are 81 years for women and 76 years for men. **Health behaviors** may explain the shorter life span in men. Men are less likely to seek care than women, are less likely to access preventive health, are more likely to consume alcohol, and overall less likely

APPLICATION OPPORTUNITY

Read back through this section and categorize the data/facts into these two categories:
Health Behaviors
Health Care Access
Would the data/facts organized in this matter be useful in gender-specific health care planning? Why or why not?

to engage in healthy lifestyle behaviors (e.g., engage in physical activity). One positive note for males is that rural male smoking behavior is declining (though not for women). And while women suffer more from depression than men, men are more likely to commit suicide.

Let's look at some specifics. According to CDC National Health Interview Survey data, more than 30% of men age 18 and over had five or more drinks in 1 day, with heavier male consumption in rural areas (CDC, 2021). This data however has sometimes not been affirmed, thus highlighting both the difficulty and variance of alcohol consumption at any given point in time or geographic location (Dixon & Chartier, 2016). Meanwhile, fewer than 50% of men exercise, but recent studies have shown the rate going up for both urban and rural men who exceed federal guidelines for exercising (WebMD, 2019). And obesity is another problem with 36% of men age 20 and over obese overall. The number is closer to 40% for rural men (Nourish by WebMD, 2018). One positive statistic shows cigarette smoking declining overall in all areas; however, rural men still smoke more than their urban counterparts (CDC, 2019).

Section Review

This section examined **gender** as one of the five elements that makes up the demographical factor. We looked at the data representing gender comparisons and the data representing comparisons rural to urban. Data and facts provided us with some insight into the gender relative to rural populations in terms of **overall health, health behaviors, and health care access**. The health behaviors and health care access differences exist when comparing women and men. Plus, rural women and men have health behaviors and health access issues that differ from their urban counterparts.

RUNNING CASE

County Health Council Grant

Meeting Agenda: Gender Focused Care Grant

Council members read the following DHHS proposal announcement:

Gender-focused care grants seek to provide needed health programs and health care services in areas often identified as needing special focus in rural areas. Examples of such special gender care gaps might include prenatal and obstetric care, education encouraging men to seek preventive services, and care for persons changing gender identity. Programs in these areas must be supported by strong demographic data and must express the growing concern of the gender-related issue in the county.

RUNNING CASE (CONTINUED)

Today's meeting focuses on reviewing the demographics of gender distribution in the county, a review of the literature on gender issues in rural communities provided by the AHEC outreach librarian, and the gender- related health resource currently available in the county. Special attention will be paid to the distribution of gender populations throughout the county and the placement of gender-related services in the county.

LEARNING ASSESSMENT—GENDER

Take this learning assessment and then compare your responses to the answers provided at the end of the book. You may find there are elements of the demographical factor you would like to review to gain a better understanding.

1. Regardless of whether women live in rural areas or urban areas, they report better health and have a longer life span than men.
   a. True
   a. False
2. Which of the following statements correctly characterize the health status of rural women compared to urban women? (Select all that apply.)
   a. Rural women report poorer health status compared to urban women.
   b. Rural women report higher unintentional injuries compared to urban women.
   c. Rural women have a higher death rate related to cardiovascular disease compared to urban women.
   d. Rural women have higher incidences of cervical cancers compared to urban women.
3. Rural women are more likely to have breast cancers diagnosed at a later stage compared to urban women. This may be associated with data that shows rural women receive _____ of the recommended screenings compared to urban women.
4. Rural women have lower rates of obesity compared to urban women.
   a. True
   b. False
5. Rural women who are pregnant are particularly placed at greater risk due to lack of health care access in rural areas. List three examples that represent this lack of health care access.

6. Shortages of mental health providers may contribute to the fact that rural women face more frequent and more violent intimate partner violence.
   a. True
   b. False

7. When comparing stroke outcomes between rural men and rural women, which of them are at a greater risk for having less favorable outcomes from strokes?

8. In addition to the shortage of mental health providers in rural areas, what other characteristics may contribute to rural women having greater occurrences of intimate partner violence? List three additional characteristics.

9. Current longevity ages are 81 years for women and 76 years for men. Select the responses that characterize health behaviors of men compared to women, which influence this life span difference. (Select all that apply.)
   a. Men are less likely to seek care than women.
   b. Men are less likely to access preventive health care than women.
   c. Men are more likely to consume alcohol than women.
   d. Men are more likely to engage in healthy lifestyle behaviors (e.g., engage in physical activity).

10. Rural male smoking behavior is declining compared to rural women.
    a. True
    b. False

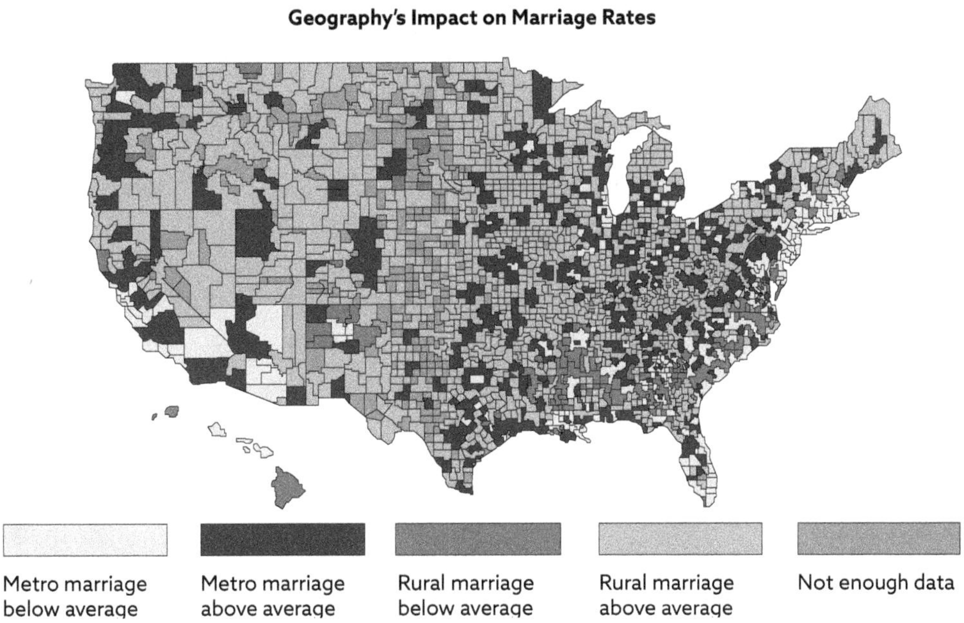

Geography's Impact on Marriage Rates

Metro marriage below average | Metro marriage above average | Rural marriage below average | Rural marriage above average | Not enough data

FIGURE 5.2   Geography's Impact on Marriage Rates.

Marital Status as an Element of the Demographical Factor

In this section we examine **marital status** as one of the five elements making up the demographical factor. There are three categories of marital status covered in the next few paragraphs. They are married, unmarried, and cohabitation. Looking at the data, we will learn that health status and health care access differ amongst these groups and also differ when comparing rural to urban. Read on to meet Martha and Henry.

Martha and Henry have been married for 29 years. High school sweethearts, they married right after graduation and parented three kids—two of which have moved away. Henry admits that he is a lot healthier than his high school classmates because Martha is so good about cooking healthy foods, dragging him for his yearly flu shot, and keeping up with his high blood pressure medicine.

Roughly 124 million were married in 2019 in a population of 331 million (Statista, 2020; USCB, 2021).This is important because repeated studies have verified that health and mortality outcomes for married persons are better than for unmarried persons. Married persons live a healthier lifestyle (e.g., exercise more, smoke less), visit doctors on a more regular basis, have lower rates of depression, have fewer strokes and heart attacks, and in general live longer (Harvard Health Publishing, 2016). Marriage, especially for men, seems to be a contributing factor to improved health outcomes. Relative to geographical distribution, nearly 51% of the rural population age 15 and older was married, compared to 44% in urban areas (Pew Research Center, 2018).

This is an interesting fact because recent trends show that persons with a higher **education** marry more than persons with lower **education**. Data from the Pew Research Center (2015) showed that 65% of persons 25 and older with a college degree were married, compared to 50% of persons with no **education** beyond high school (Pew Research Center, 2017). Rural areas do not follow this same trend. Instead, rural marriage rates are higher independent of educational attainment. Equally interesting is that rural children growing up in poor households have higher marriage rates than the national average, and they marry at a younger age and higher rate than their urban counterparts in same income households (Daily Yonder, 2017).

One cautionary note: Not all marriages have health benefits. Uncaring spouses negate the positive effects of marriage. And while divorced or single males report worse health outcomes, widowed men report worse outcomes than divorced or single men (Stahl & Schulz, 2014). Thus, it is the relationship within the marriage and the interaction of spouses that contributes to the positive health effect of marriage.

While much of the research data has focused on marriage and its health effect, less is known about the positive (or negative) impact of cohabitation. Some studies have suggested that cohabitation may not provide the permanency of marriage and may not provide the health benefits of a stable, married relationship. However, cross-cultural studies suggest that when cohabitation mirrors marriage (has longevity, has strong relationship value) then the health benefits for cohabitation share those of marriage (Perelli-Harris, 2018).

Section Review

This section examined **marital status** as one of the five elements comprising the demographical factor. We looked at the data that highlights the positive health benefit of being married, especially for men. Then we reviewed how marital status differs in rural areas (e.g., greater number of people married, younger age for marriage), while noting the effect that losing a spouse has on health outcomes. Lastly, we briefly reviewed the role of **cohabitation** and its potential health benefits.

RUNNING CASE

County Health Council Grant

Meeting Agenda: Mental Health Focus Grant

Council members read the following DHHS announcement:

The mental health grant aims to address health concerns for issues related to depression and grief counseling. DHHS acknowledges that rural communities often have higher numbers of married couples. But as these couples age, the probability of losing a spouse increases. Rural communities, which often lack mental health workers, may need assistance in sponsoring programs to address mental health concerns (e.g., grief and/or depression) associated with the loss of a spouse.

Today's meeting focuses on reviewing the demographics of married couples in the county, the age distribution of these married couples, and the health resources currently available for those who have lost a spouse.

LEARNING ASSESSMENT—MARITAL STATUS

Take this learning assessment and then compare your responses to the answers provided at the end of the book. You may find there are elements of the demographical factor you would like to review to gain a better understanding.

1. Health and mortality outcomes for married persons are better than for unmarried persons.
   a. True
   b. False

2. In general, married persons live longer than unmarried persons. List some health behaviors and health outcomes that contribute to married people living longer than unmarried people.

3. Marriage, especially for men, seems to be a contributing factor to improved health outcomes.
   a. True
   b. False

4. Rural areas do not follow the same trend for marriage rates and educational attainment as urban areas. Instead rural marriages rates are higher independent of educational attainment. What data supports this assertion?

5. Rural children growing up in poor households have rates lower than the national average to marry and to marry at a younger age and lower than their urban counterparts in same income households.

6. Cross-cultural studies suggest that when cohabitation mirrors marriage (has longevity, has strong relationship value), the health benefits for cohabitation share those of marriage.
   a. True
   b. False

Education Level as an Element of the Demographical Factor

The last of the five elements constituting the demographical factor is **Education** level. We will take a look at data that demonstrating that education attainment impacts **life style choices** as well as **health care access** and **health outcomes**. Let's meet James to help understand why education level matters (see the box on this page).

James is a third-generation Pikesvillian. His grandfather started a small home repair business that James's dad turned into a residential and commercial construction business. For as long as James can remember, he has been helping in the family business—first filing invoices in the office, then when he turned 16, hauling construction waste to the dump. Upon graduation from high school, James moved full time into the business often working alongside his dad and older brother.

Education has been associated with improved health outcomes, longer life spans, and greater utilization of preventive services. By some estimates those with a high school degree live longer than those without such a degree often as much as 4 years (U.S. Depart. of Health and Human Services, 2012), and those with a college degree live by as much as five years longer that those who hold a high school diploma or do not finish high school. Why is this? Some studies suggest that the more educated adopt healthier lifestyles. For instance, less than 13% of those with a college degree smoke, compared with 30% of high school graduates. Other studies have shown that college graduates are more likely to exercise and make better food selections. Most rank their health as good or very good. In fact, across ethnic/racial groups, the less the educational attainment the greater the percentage of respondents that rank their health as less than good. Moreover, educational attainment and health outcomes link not only to adults but to children as well. Children of parents who have not attained a high school degree are more likely to be in poor or fair health than children with parents who have obtained more education (RWJ Foundation, 2009).

Nationally, nearly 36% of the population have a 4-year degree or higher. The vast majority (by some estimates as many as 90% of college graduates) live/work in urban/suburban areas. The remaining 10% of college graduates reside in rural areas. However, this data could be misleading as there are more persons overall living in urban/suburban areas than in rural areas. Instead, determining percentage of persons with college degree by population density of the area finds the numbers are closer together. And the trend for obtaining more education mirrors this percentage increase for both geographical areas. An interesting fact is that there may be greater variation in the percentage of rural citizens with a college degree between various rural areas than between rural and urban areas. That is college attainment. Does high school attainment follow similar lines?

Nationally, 83% graduate from high school in four years (2015 data). This compares to a graduation rate of 87% of high school students in rural areas who graduate within 4 years. Thus, it would appear that rural students graduate at higher rates than their urban counterparts (Showalter et. al., 2017). For the most part this is true; however, students of color in rural areas had lower graduation rates (77%) than their White, non-Hispanic classmates—and this a slightly

> **APPLICATION OPPORTUNITY**
>
> View this interactive map to see rates of college degree attainment by geography https://s3.amazonaws.com/interactives.americanprogress.org/maps/2018/12/Adult+Attainment+Report/index.html

> **Education** has been defined by Robert Wood Johnson as "educational attainment, or the years or level of overall schooling a person has, rather than instruction on specific health topics like hygiene, diet or exercise" (Robert Wood Johnson Foundation, 2011).

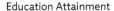

Education Attainment

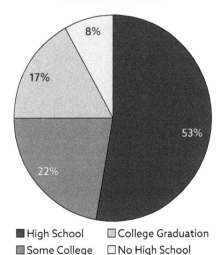

- 53%
- 8%
- 17%
- 22%

■ High School ☐ College Graduation
■ Some College ☐ No High School

After several years of working as a general contractor in the business, James decided to go to the local community college to obtain an HVAC certificate. This allowed him to carry heating units previously unavailable to the firm. When the electrician at the business retired 4 years earlier, James went back to the college, enrolling in an electrician course and ultimately obtaining an electrician license. This allowed the business to be assured that a licensed electrician was signing off on the work they did.

APPLICATION OPPORTUNITY

Collect and apply data: Look at data profiles for your county. How does this data compare to state and national data? Is there data that could be underreported, if so explain.

lower graduation rate than persons of color nationally. Within rural communities, rural women are better educated than rural men, with women holding proportionately more degrees at all educational levels (The 74, 2017). This is consistent with national rural education trends.

Another difference within rural communities appears across ages. Younger rural residents under 25 have higher graduation rates and educational attainments than older rural residents. Of key importance is the variation of high school graduation rates between rural areas, with poorer counties falling below both the national and state averages for graduation rates.

One caveat relative to educational level data is the multiple ways it is presented. For instance, one might see a pie chart like the one on the next page.

A quick look might lead someone to say that the high school completion rate is 53%, when in fact the high school completion rate is 92% (53% completed high school, 22% completed high school and went on to do some college work, and 17% completed high school and went on to graduate from college). If stating the percentage of those that only completed high school, 53% would be correct.

Another often misinterpreted statistics is presented as such:

At Least High School Graduate	78.5%
At Least Bachelor's Degree	11.6%

While this accurately identifies those who have attained at least a high school diploma, the numbers underrepresent educational attainment in the county. For this, let's return to James (see the box on this page).

We see through James's experience that educational attainment may ebb and flow and the presence in a community of a local community college is critical. As of 2013, roughly 50% of the 1,200 community colleges were in rural areas (Rural Community College Alliance; Science Foundation AZ). These colleges provide trades education, stepping-stone programs to 4-year institutions, and serve as a continuous educational reservoir for residents needing workforce development, enrichment, and new skills. Unfortunately, some statistical reporting of participation in or graduation from community college programs is unidentified in some county level data profiles. You must look carefully to ensure that the database you are using presents the best educational picture for your county.

Section Review

In this section we looked at a fifth element of the demographical factor, the element **educational level** and the impact on rural **health care access**. A significant correlate to improved **health outcomes** and **lifestyle choices**, educational attainment was reviewed relative to urban–rural differences and within rural populations (age differences, gender differences in age attainment). Lastly, we caution the need to look closely at educational data presentation as misinterpretations can occur when only considering a cursory view of the data.

RUNNING CASE

County Health Council Grant

Meeting Agenda: Obesity Prevention and Nutritious Living Grant

Council members read the following grant proposal:

DHHS continues to be concerned about the growing rate of obesity across all age demographics. Interested in finding programs to address obesity prevention through more nutritious living, communities are encouraged to apply for funds to find new ways to develop educational material that impacts the obesity rates in their county. Counties must demonstrate that programs developed are consistent with the educational and interest level of their citizens.

Today's meeting focuses on reviewing the education distribution in the county, the relationship between health literacy and education, and the health outcome statistics for obesity in the county.

LEARNING ASSESSMENT—EDUCATION LEVEL

Take this learning assessment and then compare your responses to the answers provided at the end of the book. You may find there are elements of the demographical factor you would like to review to gain a better understanding.

1. Education has been associated with _____ health outcomes, _____ life spans, and _____ utilization of preventive services.

2. Person with a high school degree live longer than those without such a degree, often as much as 4 years.
   a. True
   b. False

3. Children of parents who have not attained a high school degree experience the same health outcomes as children with parents who have obtained more education.
   a. True
   b. False

4. When comparing rural-to-urban education data, such as percentage of people with college degrees, consideration should be made for population density. Explain how to calculate population density (see Chapter 2). Why would population density be relevant to understanding educational data?

5. Students of color in rural areas have _____ graduation rates than their White, non-Hispanic classmates and _____ graduation rates than persons of color nationally.

6. Within rural communities, rural women are less educated than rural men, with men holding proportionately more degrees at all educational levels.
   a. True
   b. False

7. These colleges provide trades education, stepping-stone programs to 4-year institutions, and serve as a continuous educational reservoir for residents needing _____ development, enrichment, and _____ _____ development.

RUNNING CASE

County Health Council Grant

Culmination of five grant meetings:

You are to play the role of a council member. Consider the agendas for the five grant meetings. Go through each week's issue/question and identify critical issues posed by the week's agenda. Support your claims with data. Rank your highest priority, and give a recommendation on how to present the information to DHHS.

CHAPTER SUMMARY

In this chapter, we explored the demographical factor highlighting key information relative to the five demographical factor elements of **age**, **race/ethnicity**, **gender**, **marital status**, and **education level**. Fortunately, there is a wealth of information about the impact that these five elements have on health outcomes. Less numerous are studies that look at the differences of how these five elements present in rural–urban areas, or the outcomes that might emerge because of rural–urban dissimilarities Nevertheless, we explored differences that do arise. We also tried to keep in mind that behind all the figures and statistics are human beings who must be remembered and factored into any health equations. As we end the chapter, you should review the Community Assessment Grid that pertains to data relevant to these five demographical elements. You might want to use the Grid in combination with the running case of the county panel members. Or you might want to craft a narrative about individuals who fit each of the demographical factor elements. In so doing, you will reinforce the reality that the numbers are really about people who comprise the data.

Using your county or a selected county, complete the Demographical Factor Assessment Grid. Be sure to populate each element with comprehensive data elements. Include all sources from which data was obtained.

TABLE 5.1 Demographical Factor County Assessment Grid Template

Factor	Elements	County Data	State Data
Demographical Factor			
	Age	Provide data regarding age distribution groups or ranges reported for county. (% of population)	
	Ethnicity	Provide data to identify ethnic groups that comprise county. (% of population)	
	Gender	Provide data regarding male compared to female as a percentage of population.	

TABLE 5.1 Demographical Factor County Assessment Grid Template *(continued)*

Factor	Elements	County Data	State Data
	Marital Status	Provide county data pertaining to marital status in county.	
		Percentage married.	
		Percentage divorced or widowed.	
		Percentage single.	
	Education Level	Provide data describing educational attainment in county.	
		Percentage with high school education.	
		Percentage with some college.	
		Percentage college graduates.	
		Percentage no high school.	

CHAPTER ACTIVITY—LEARNING CHALLENGE

Below are two learning challenges designed to help apply the demographical factor's elements in a systematic review. The learning challenges can be completed individually or in a small group.

Learning Challenge 1: Fayetteville is a rural, 14,000-person community attracting many retirees from neighboring metro areas. Several health systems have initiated discussions with the local 250-bed general hospital about a potential partnership. Critical to the discussions are the health resources of the area compared to this growing trend in retirees.

a. What health care resources might be anticipated for a county with a growing retiree population?

b. Discuss how the health care needs of this elderly population may be more complex if within this population there is a high percentage of widowed or single elderly. What might these two demographic characteristics imply for the kind of health services to be provided soon in Fayetteville?

Learning Challenge 2: Thomas is a 30-year-old African American male and a veteran who lives near Jackson, which is a rural community of 35,000 primarily composed of farmers and ranchers. Thomas works as a mechanic in a small automobile repair shop.

   a. Identify the three demographic elements describing Thomas in this scenario, and discuss how these three demographic elements may impact his health status.
   b. Based on these three demographic elements, how might his access to health care be impacted?

CHAPTER ACTIVITY—PRACTICE VIGNETTES

Below are three practice vignettes. Read the scenario and answer the questions following each scenario. These practice vignettes may be completed individually or in small groups.

Vignette 1: Tenisha, a 35-year-old woman, met her husband shortly after graduating from Shaw University. They both were lucky to find jobs in Raleigh where he worked as a manager for a large investment firm and she worked as an assistant director for an arts nonprofit. Then the children came, and Tenisha became a full- time mom. But now, following a messy bankruptcy and an even messier divorce, Tenisha has decided to move back home to Bath to be near her parents, sister, and family friends. But she is worried. Even though Tenisha has a college degree in history, she is not sure about finding working to support herself and her two children, 10-year-old Wesley and 12-year-old Faith.

   a. Given that Tenisha is a single mom, how would her gender and marital status affect/ predict her health care usage?
   b. Discuss the impact that Tenisha's educational level has on health care decisions for herself and her children.

Vignette 2: Silvia is about the finish her physician assistant studies. She is considering moving to a rural community and has begun exploring [name a hometown in your state of less than 40,000 people]. To aid in her decision-making, she has drawn a 30-mile radius around the town and is exploring the kind of health care practices/facilities that exist there, as well as the kind of medical insurance prevalent in the area.

   a. What is the population and race/ethnic distribution in the county? How does this compare to state statistics?
   b. Explain how demographic statistics you just provided might impact health care needs in the county.

Vignette 3: [name a town of less than 20,000 residents with retirement amenities] is a rural community attracting many retirees from neighboring cities. Several health systems have initiated discussions with the local hospital about a potential partnership. Critical to the discussions are the health resources of the area compared to the demographic data.

a. What health care resources should be anticipated for a county with a large population of retirees?

b. Discuss how the health care needs of this elderly population may be more complex if within this population there is a high percentage of widowed or single elderly. What might these two demographic characteristics imply for the kind of health services to be provided?

REFERENCES—AGE

Baernholdt, M., Yan, G., Hinton, I., Rose, K., & Mattos, M. (2012). Quality of life in rural and urban adults 65 years and older: Findings from the national health and nutrition examination survey. *The Journal of Rural Health, 28*(4), 339–347. doi:10.1111/j.1748-0361.2011.00403.x

Centers for Disease Control and Prevention. (2017, September 22). Child health in rural America. https://www.cdc.gov/ruralhealth/child-health.html

Georgetown University Health Policy Institute Center for Children and Families, (2017 October 20). Research update: Health care in rural and urban America. https://ccf.georgetown.edu/2017/10/20/research-update-health-care-in-rural-and-urban-america/

Kelleher, K. J., & Gardner, W. (2017). Out of sight, out of mind — behavioral and developmental care for rural children. *The New England Journal of Medicine, 376*(14), 1301–1303. doi:10.1056/NEJMp1700713

North Carolina Health News. (November 18, 2019). Rural-urban divide continues to widen, reports finds. https://www.northcarolinahealthnews.org/2019/11/18/rural-urban-divide-widens-cdc-finds/

Pew Research Center (May 22, 2018). Demographic and economic trends in urban, suburban and rural communities. https://www.pewresearch.org/social-trends/2018/05/22/demographic-and-economic-trends-in-urban-suburban-and-rural-communities

Probst, J. C., Barker, J. C., Enders, A., & Gardiner, P. (2018). Current state of child health in rural America: How context shapes children's health. *The Journal of Rural Health, 34*(S1), s3–s12. doi:10.1111/jrh.12222

Rural Health Leaders. (2016, April 20). Rural children face steep healthcare challenges. https://www.healthleadersmedia.com/strategy/rural-children-face-steep-healthcare-challenges

Rural Health Research. (2019, August). Healthcare access and status among rural children. https://www.ruralhealthresearch.org/recaps/9

Rural Information Hub. (2018). Rural Aging. https://www.ruralhealthinfo.org/topics/aging

U.S. Census Bureau. (December 8, 2016). New Census data show differences between urban and rural populations. https://www.census.gov/newsroom/press-releases/2016/cb16-210.html

United States Department of Agriculture. (2018, November). Rural America at a glance, 2018 edition. https://www.ers.usda.gov/webdocs/publications/90556/eib200_brochureformat.pdf?v=5899.2

REFERENCES—RACE/ETHNICITY

Centers for Disease Control and Prevention. (November 17, 2017). Racial/ethnic health disparities among rural adults—United States, 2012–2015. https://www.cdc.gov/mmwr/volumes/66/ss/ss6623a1.htm

CDC Vital Signs. (2015, May). Hispanic health. https://www.cdc.gov/vitalsigns/hispanic-health/index.html

Economic Research Service—U.S. Department of Agriculture. (n.d.). Racial and ethnic diversity is increasing in America [graphic]. https://www.ers.usda.gov/webdocs/publications/44331/10597_page7.pdf?v=41055

Economic Research Service—U.S. Department of Agriculture. (October 13, 2020). Racial and ethnic minorities made up about 22 percent of the rural population in 2018, compared to 43 percent in urban areas. https://www.ers.usda.gov/data-products/chart-gallery/gallery/chart-detail/?chartId=99538

Health Resources and Services Administration, Office of Health Equity. (2018). Health equity report 2017. United States Department of Health and Human Services. https://www.hrsa.gov/sites/default/files/hrsa/health-equity/2017-HRSA-health-equity-report.pdf

Housing Assistance Rural Research Brief. (2012, April). Race & ethnicity in rural America. http://www.ruralhome.org/storage/research_notes/rrn-race-and-ethnicity-web.pdf

James, C., Moonesinghe, R., Wilson-Frederick, S., Hall, J., Penman-Aguilar, A., & Bouye, K. (2017). Racial/ethnic health disparities among rural adults—United States, 2012–2015. *Morbidity and Mortality Weekly Report: Surveillance Summaries, 66*(23), 1–9. Retrieved May 28, 2021, from https://www.jstor.org/stable/26403139

Musa, D., Schulz, R., Harris, R., Silverman, M., & Thomas, S. B. (2009). Trust in the health care system and the use of preventive health services by older black and white adults. *American Journal of Public Health*, 99(7), 1293–1299. https://doi.org/10.2105/AJPH.2007.123927

Pew Research Center. (2015, June 11). Multiracial in America. https://www.pewsocialtrends.org/2015/06/11/multiracial-in-america/

Probst, J. C., Moore, C. G., Glover, S. H., & Samuels, M. E. (2004). Person and place: The compounding effects of race/ethnicity and rurality on health. *American Journal of Public Health, 94*(10), 1695–1703. doi:10.2105/AJPH.94.10.1695

The Commonwealth Fund. (January 14, 2021). Understanding and ameliorating medical mistrust among Black Americans. https://www.commonwealthfund.org/publications/ newsletter-article/2021/jan/medical-mistrust-among-black-americans

The Hill. (August 24, 2017). Black Americans don't trust our healthcare system—here's why. https://thehill.com/blogs/pundits-blog/healthcare/347780-black-americans-dont-have-trust-in-our-healthcare-system).

United States Department of Agriculture. (2012, April). Rural America at a glance, 2018—Population trends vary by race/ethnicity. https://www.ers.usda.gov/webdocs/publications/90556/ eib200_brochureformat.pdf

U.S. Department of Health and Human Services—Office of Minority Health (n.d.) Profile: Black/ African Americans. https://www.minorityhealth.hhs.gov/omh/browse.aspx?lvl=3&lvlid=61

REFERENCES—GENDER

Barefoot, K. N., Warren, J. C., & Smalley, K. B. (2017). Women's health care: The experiences and behaviors of rural and urban lesbians in the USA. *Rural and Remote Health, 17*(1), 3875.

Centers for Disease Control and Prevention. (November 25, 2019). Tobacco use by geographic region. https://www.cdc.gov/tobacco/disparities/geographic/index.htm

Centers for Disease Control and Prevention. (April 14, 2021). Men's health. https://www.cdc .gov/nchs/fastats/mens-health.htm

Cepeda-Benito, A., Doogan, N. J., Redner, R., Roberst, M. E., Kurti, A. N., Villanti, A. C., Lopez, A.A., Quisenberry, A.J., Stanton, C.A., Gaalema, D.E., Keith, D.R., Parker, M.A., & Higgins, S. T. (2018). Trend differences in men and women in rural and urban U.S. settings. *Preventative Medicine, 117,* 69–75. https://www.sciencedirect.com/science/article/ pii/S0091743518301191

Committee opinion no. 586: Health disparities in rural women. (2014). *Obstetrics & Gynecology, 123*(2, PART 1), 384–388. doi:10.1097/01.AOG.0000443278.06393.d6

Dixon, M. A., & Chartier, K. G. (2016). Alcohol use patterns among urban and rural residents: demographic and social influences. *Alcohol Research: Current Reviews, 38*(1), 69–77.

Nourish by WebMD. (June 19, 2018). Obesity plagues rural America. https://www.webmd .com/diet/obesity/news/20180619/obesity-plagues-rural-america#1

Health Resources and Service Administration. (2010). Women's health USA 2010. https://mchb. hrsa.gov/whusa10/popchar/pages/110ruw.html

Illinois Department of Public Health Men's Health. (n.d.). Why's men's health? http://www .idph.state.il.us/menshealth/

Lewis, C., Paxton, I., & Zephyrin, L. (2019, August 15). The rural maternity health crisis. *The Commonwealth Fund.* https://www.commonwealthfund.org/blog/2019/rural-maternity-care-crisis

Medical News Today. (May 27, 2021). Which women are most at risk of stroke? https://www.medicalnewstoday.com/articles/320867

National Rural Health Association. (2013). National Rural Health Association Policy Brief: Rural women's health. https://www.ruralhealthweb.org/advocate/policy-documents

National Vital Statistics. (2019, June 24). United States life tables 2017 https://www.cdc.gov/nchs/data/nvsr/nvsr68/nvsr68_07-508.pdf

Nguyen-Pham, S., BDSc, Leung, J., BHS, & McLaughlin, D., PhD. (2014). Disparities in breast cancer stage at diagnosis in urban and rural adult women: A systematic review and meta-analysis. *Annals of Epidemiology, 24*(3), 228–235. doi:10.1016/j.annepidem.2013.12.002

Peek-Asa, C., Wallis, A., Harland, K., Beyer, K., Dickey, P., & Saftlas, A. (2011). Rural disparity in domestic violence prevalence and access to resources. *Journal of Women's Health, 20*(11), 1743–1749. https://doi.org/10.1089/jwh.2011.2891

Pew Research Center. (2018, June 19). Family life is changing in different ways across urban, suburban and rural communities in the U.S. https://www.pewresearch.org/fact-tank/2018/06/19/family-life-is-changing-in-different-ways-across-urban-suburban-and-rural-communities-in-the-u-s/

Steelesmith D. L., Fontanella, C. A., Campo J. V., Bridge J. A., Warren K. L., & Root E. D. (2019). Contextual factors associated with county-level suicide rates in the United States, 1999 to 2016. *JAMA Netw Open, 2*(9), e1910936. doi:10.1001/jamanetworkopen.2019.10936

United States Census Bureau. (2017, August 9). One in five Americans live in rural areas. https://www.census.gov/library/stories/2017/08/rural-america.html

United States Census Bureau. (2019). QuickFacts. https://www.census.gov/quickfacts/fact/table/IN,US/LFE046218

United States Department of Health and Human Services, Health Resources and Services Administration, Maternal and Child Health Bureau. (2013). Women's health USA 2013. https://mchb.hrsa.gov/whusa13/population-characteristics/p/rural-urban-women.html

WebMD. (2019, June 13). CDC: Exercise rates up for urban, rural Americans. https://www.webmd.com/fitness-exercise/news/20190613/cdc-exercise-rates-up-for-urban-rural-americans#1

REFERENCES—MARITAL STATUS

Daily Yonder. (2017, August 26). Rural upbringing increase odds that young people will marry. https://www.dailyyonder.com/rural-upbringing-increases-odds-young-people-will-mary/2017/08/16/

Harvard Health Publishing Harvard Medical School. (2016, November 30). The health advantages of marriage. https://www.health.harvard.edu/blog/the-health-advantages-of-marriage-2016113010667

Harvard Health Publishing Harvard Medical School. (2019, June 5). Marriage and men's health. https://www.health.harvard.edu/mens-health/marriage-and-mens-health

Perelli-Harris, B., Hoherz, S., Addo, F., Lappegård, T., Evans, A., Sassler, S., & Styrc, M. (2018). Do marriage and cohabitation provide benefits to health in mid-life? The role of childhood selection mechanisms and partnership characteristics across countries. *Population Research and Policy Review*, 37(5), 703–728. https://doi.org/10.1007/s11113-018-9467-3

Pew Research Center. (2017, September 14). As U.S. marriage rates hovers at 50% education gap in marital status widens. https://www.pewresearch.org/fact-tank/2017/09/14/as-u-s-marriage-rate-hovers-at-50-education-gap-in-marital-status-widens/

Pew Research Center. (2018, June 19). Family life is changing in different ways across urban, suburban and rural communities in the U.S. https://www.pewresearch.org/fact-tank/2018/06/19/family-life-is-changing-in-different-ways-across-urban-suburban-and-rural-communities-in-the-u-s/

Robert Wood Johnson Foundation Commission to Build a Healthier America. (Sept. 2009). Education matters for health. [pdf]. http://www.commissiononhealth.org/PDF/c270deb3-ba42-4fbd-baeb-2cd65956f00e/Issue%20Brief%206%20Sept%2009%20-%20Education%20and%20Health.pdf

Robards, J., Evandrou, M., Falkingham, J., & Vlachantoni, A. (2012). Marital status, health and mortality. *Maturitas*, 73(4), 295–299. doi:10.1016/j.maturitas.2012.08.007

Stahl, S. T., & Schulz, R. (2014). The effect of widowhood on husbands' and wives' physical activity: the Cardiovascular Health Study. *Journal of Behavioral Medicine*, 37(4), 806–817. https://doi.org/10.1007/s10865-013-9532-7

REFERENCES—EDUCATION LEVEL

The 74. (2017, June 1). Solving the rural education gap: Weigh in on new report's findings tying gap to prosperity. https://www.the74million.org/article/solving-the-rural-education-gap-experts-weigh-in-on-new-reports-findings-tying-gap-to-prosperity/

Bolin, J. N., Bellamy, G. R., Ferdinand, A. O., Vuong, A. M., Kash, B. A., Schulze, A., & Helduser, J. W. (2015). Rural healthy people 2020: New decade, same challenges. *The Journal of Rural Health*, 31(3), 326–333. doi:10.1111/jrh.12116

CityLab. (2018, October 31). The talent dividend in urban and rural areas. https://www.citylab.com/life/2018/10/college-education-workforce-urban-rural-divide-jobs/574273/

Robert Wood Johnson Foundation. (2011, April 11). Education and health. https://www.rwjf.org/en/library/research/2011/05/education-matters-for-health.html

Rural Community College Alliance.(n.d.) Creating opportunities in place. https://ruralccalliance.org

Science Foundation Arizona. (n.d.). Making a difference: Community colleges are key drivers of rural development. http://www.sfaz.org/making-difference-community-colleges-key-drivers-rural-development

Showalter, D., Klein, R., Johnson, J., & Hartman, S. L. (2017, June). Why rural matters 2015–2016: Understanding the landscape. [pdf]. http://www.ruraledu.org/user_uploads/file/WRM-2015-16.pdf

Statista. (2021). Number of married couples in the United States from 1960 to 2020. https://www.statista.com/statistics/183663/number-of-married-couples-in-the-us/

U.S. Census Bureau. (May 27, 2021). U.S. and world population clock. https://www.census.gov/popclock/

United States Department of Health and Human Services. (2012). [pdf]. Health, United States, 2011 with special feature on socioeconomic status and health. https://www.cdc.gov/nchs/data/hus/hus11.pdf

Figure Credits

IMG 5.0: Copyright © 2016 Depositphotos/Rawpixel.

Fig. 5.1: Source: https://www.ers.usda.gov/data-products/chart-gallery/gallery/chart-detail/?chartId=99538.

Fig. 5.2: Daily Yonder, "Geography's Impact on Marriage Rates," https://www.dailyyonder.com/rural-upbringing-increases-odds-young-people-will-mary/2017/08/16/20875/. Copyright © 2017 by Center for Rural Strategies.

Chapter Six

The Support Factor

Introduction

In this chapter we explore the fifth factor of the Rural Health Framework: the support factor. As we know, support comes in many ways: financial support, programmatic, legislative or regulatory. Support may also come from agencies or groups whose mission is to inform policy makers, influencers, or investors. Support comes from local, state, or national entities and may focus on a population or geographical area. In this chapter we will delve into five elements that comprise the support factor: local governance, federal agencies, national programs/organizations, telehealth, and health interventions.

The running case in this chapter also serves to highlight the resources available to professionals who choose to practice in rural health or provide resources to rural areas. Lastly, this chapter has a different focus than previous chapters. Instead of looking at comparisons between urban and rural or the manifestation of health outcomes, we start with the premise that rural areas require special attention because of poor health outcomes and ongoing needs. This may result from a lack of knowledge or focus on the part of legislators and policy makers who more often reside in urban areas and are thus more familiar with those areas. It may be due to laws and regulations being enacted to impact the largest number of people, which often means that people living in rural areas may not have as much influence on legal and policy outcomes. It also means that rural

Learning Outcomes

After reading about the support factor, the learner will be able to

- Identify the five elements that make up the support factor.

- Explain how each of the elements impact the health status and/or health care access of people living in rural areas.

- Analyze and apply the support factor and the elements constituting the support factor by assessing their contribution to rural health outcomes.

Key Topics

Learning about the following key topics will support you in achieving the chapter outcomes:

- **Local Governance:**
  local boards of health, county commissioners
- **Federal Agencies:**
  the Centers for Disease Control (CDC), the Office of Rural Health Policy (FORHP), the Rural Health Research Center Program, and the Office of Rural Mental Health Research (ORMHR)
- **National Programs/Organizations:**
  Area Health Education Centers (AHECs), County Health Rankings, Cooperative Extension Service (CES), national organizations
- **Telehealth:**
  telemedicine, telepsychiatry, telepharmacy
- **Rural Health Interventions:**
  health centers, expanded roles

issues are complex and require focused attention. Thus, this chapter does not seek to compare the support vehicles between urban and rural; instead, the chapter explores specific support elements that are found in and focused on rural health concerns.

RUNNING CASE

Ms. Jones's Health Science Class

Ms. Jones, the health sciences teacher for Rural County High School, wants to expand her health care workforce curriculum. She has, therefore, invited several other high school teachers as well as a few community members to help her think through how best to help her students broaden their perspective of health careers and find resources should they wish to pursue a health career.

Local Governance as an Element of the Support Factor

Policy formulation, regulatory initiatives, and funding all occur as much at the local as at the national level. In this section, we want to explore several local entities that provide support resources to local health concerns and issues. Specially, we will review local boards of health and county commissioners.

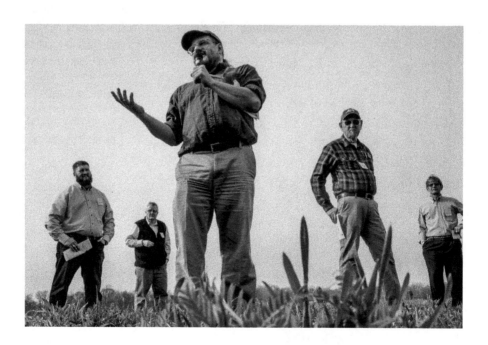

LOCAL BOARDS OF HEALTH

Boards of health have a long tradition in the United States. For instance, in 1799, Paul Revere was chairman of the Board of Health in Boston, the first local health board in Massachusetts. He and his fellow board members were given broad authority to control the "filth and offal" that contaminated the environment and produced deadly epidemics. Since their creation, local boards of health have had as their mission to help promote, protect, and improve the health of the residents within the jurisdiction of the board. Local boards of health have also embraced protection of environmental as well as public health (Massachusetts Association of Health Boards, n.d.).

> **APPLICATION OPPORTUNITY**
>
> For an interesting perspective on the tension between national and state boards of health, see the following website: https://www.ncbi.nlm.nih.gov/pmc/articles/PMC3001811/.

For the most part, local boards of health are community members—with Department of Public Health representatives—who perform a variety of duties. Boards of health are policy making bodies that help to draft policies, guidelines, recommendations, and opinions about a broad range of health concerns (e.g., smoking in public places, concealed weapons, soda tax). As an example, the Board of Health in Kent County, Michigan, has tackled such issues as banning trans fats in restaurants, regulating e-cigarettes, and requiring the use of bicycle helmets (AccessKent Kent County Michigan, n.d.).

> **APPLICATION OPPORTUNITY**
>
> Boards of health may encompass different geographical areas or jurisdictions. Compare duties/roles of county health boards, district boards of health, public health authority boards, and/or consolidated human services boards.

Local boards of health can be charged with oversight of the local public health department. For instance, this oversight could include the hiring and evaluation of the public health director. Local boards of health can also adopt and revise rules and regulations pertaining to the administration of public health laws (Tri-County Health Department, n.d.). In addition to policy and oversight responsibilities, most Boards of Health are involved in assessing community health needs, assisting with workforce development, serving as a liaison with other local entities or state agencies, and serving as a community voice in the design and implementation of public health programs (Iowa Department of Public Health, 2018).

COUNTY COMMISSIONERS

Next, we will discuss the role of **county commissioners** as form of local governance. We are using the title **county commissioner** because most states use this title at this level of local

County commissioners are decision-makers in regards to health care in rural counties. Read here about New Hanover County Hospital: https://portcitydaily.com/story/2020/07/11/new-hanover-commissioners-to-vote-on-next-nhrmc-sale-step-big-financial-questions-remain/

governance. The requirements for being a county commissioner may vary by state, but for our discussion we will cover the most common requirements for **county commissioners**. First, commissioners run for the office and are elected by voting held in the county where they are to serve. They must reside in the county, making county commissioners well known to the residents where they live and work—they may be a teacher at the local school, a nurse at the local hospital, a farmer, or a homemaker. **County commissioners** have a vested interest in the betterment of their county (Byers, 2008).

While **county commissioner** positions are budgeted and they are paid as part-time employees, the realty is they are always on duty. People from their district may call at any time of the day or night to voice a concern. When commissioners are out in public shopping or attending church, people in the community approach them to ask for their help and influence in addressing local issues. The concerns may vary from farmland being converted to a solar farm to expanding the hours at the landfill to accommodate local residents.

Their role requires they attend regularly scheduled commissioner meetings and community events. As we discovered that festivals make up an important part of the sociocultural factor of rural areas, one would expect to see their **county commissioner** in attendance at these events. Also, the **county commissioner** would attend the opening celebrations for new businesses and be involved at some level with attracting businesses to the area.

Aside from knowing the residents of the county and their concerns, **county commissioners** also build relationships with the people serving in county departments. Establishing and maintaining effective relationships with other county officials and personnel is essential for commissioners' ability to represent the concerns of residents. Conversely, commissioners help to communicate with and educate residents about upcoming changes in the county. Perhaps home and hospice care had been a services provided by the health department but are being eliminated, instead allowing home health and hospice services to be offered to the community through a private provider. Since **county commissioners** would have participated in making such decisions, they are well suited for educating and informing residents.

APPLICATION OPPORTUNITY

Go to the website of the county where you reside and find the names of your county commissioners. Do you know any of these **county commissioners**?

Section Review

In this section we have looked at local governance as the first element comprising the support factor. Specifically, we discussed the roles of local boards of health and county commissioners, along with how their influence impacts the health and well-being of rural residents. We introduced Ms. Jones, a health science teacher, who is expanding her students' knowledge of potential health careers. Now we have begun with this chapter to recognize the support systems that impact health outcomes in rural areas.

LEARNING ASSESSMENT—LOCAL GOVERNANCE

Take this learning assessment and then compare your responses to the answers provided at the end of the book. You may find there are elements of the support factor you would like to review to gain a better understanding.

1. List the five elements comprising the support factor.
2. Local boards of health protect the public health and also environmental health.
   a. True
   b. False
3. List example examples of the oversight that local boards of health have in regard to the health department.
4. County commissioners are appointed by the state governor.
   a. True
   b. False
5. Give three examples of what county commissioners do to serve their county.

Federal Agencies as an Element of the Support Factor

Rural health has significantly poor health outcomes, which draw the attention of federal policy makers. Perhaps because so many legislators come from urban areas and lack first-hand experience with rural issues or because legislatures respond to the largest cohort of constituents, who are usually situated in urban areas, policy makers commission and fund specific agencies to track rural health data and rural issues. In this second element in the support factor—the **federal agency** element—we will explore several key agencies devoted to improving rural health.

CENTERS FOR DISEASE CONTROL AND PREVENTION (CDC)

As the national health center, the CDC has broad authority for monitoring and informing policy makers, practitioners, and the public relative to the health of the American people. Within the CDC, rural health is highlighted for special attention. Sometimes that focus takes the form of a special report series such as the 2017 series. More commonly, the CDC reports on health issues in rural America through its Rural Health Section. These issues might be disease specific (that is, COPD, cancer) or special focus areas in rural America such as suicide rates, antibiotic usage, or vaccination.

Equally as important as reporting the health data, the CDC describes "success stories" of interventions in rural areas that have improved health access and overall health outcomes in rural areas. These success stories range from an asthma intervention by the Montana Department of Public Health and Human Services, to the Kentucky Department of Health's arthritis program to Michigan's "Be a Disease Detective" geared toward 4-H youth. These success stories help to distribute information about innovative programs and in so doing both reward innovation and encourage others to focus on rural health programs in their communities.

THE FEDERAL OFFICE OF RURAL HEALTH POLICY (FORHP)

The Federal Office of Rural Health Policy is charged "with advising the Secretary of the U.S. Department of Health and Human Services on the effect that federal health care policies and regulations may have on rural community" (Health Resources & Services Administration, 2019). The Office also provides funding to local communities to increase access to care and improve health of rural populations (Health Resources & Services Administration, 2020). Sample projects funded by FORHP include the Black Lung Clinics Program, small health care provider quality improvement program, and radiation exposure screening and education program, to name just a few. FORHP has four main programs designed to increase access to care for rural populations. These programs are the Community Based Division (CBD), Hospital State Division (HSD), Office for the Advancement of Telehealth (OAT), and the Policy Research Division (PRD).

THE RURAL HEALTH RESEARCH CENTER PROGRAM

The Rural Health Research Center is funded by the federal government to produce policy-relevant research on health care and population health in rural areas. Throughout the country, there are 10 funded Research Centers, each with specific areas of expertise or focus. The Research Centers award research projects aimed at improving health outcomes, meeting the needs of the Federal Office of Rural Health, and providing evidence-based outcomes that might transfer to other areas. Projects funded through Rural Health Research Centers include activities of a rural hospital and the impacts of initiating specialized care in these hospitals. Some past projects have included loss of obstetric care in rural hospitals, cancer prevention and control activities in rural hospitals, and changes in services offered by rural hospitals. Projects also track demographics (elders in rural areas and services provided and needed), funding impacts on rural hospitals (Medicare payments and adjustments for geographic cost differences), and data collection of rural health-related measures (standards of care, mental health trends, telemedicine, opioid prescriptions trends in rural Medicare populations), to name just a few. Data obtained from the Rural Health Research Centers informs regional and national organizations and individuals seeking to understand and improve policy and administrative programs in rural areas.

THE OFFICE OF RURAL MENTAL HEALTH RESEARCH (ORMHR)

The Office of Rural Mental Health Research is mandated by Congress to coordinate the research activities of the Department of Health and Human Services related to the mental health of residents in rural areas and to coordinate and synergize health and human services activities with critical related activities of public and nonprofit entities (National Institute of Mental Health, 2018). Among the various activities that the office sponsors are webinars open to the public. For instance, in their 2018 webinar series titled Mental Health and Rural America: Challenges and Opportunities, presenters from multiple disciplines described the unique needs of rural populations relative to mental health services and resources. Programs such as these help to inform, activate, and disseminate findings gathered through other programs and research initiatives (National Institute of Mental Health, 2018).

> **APPLICATION OPPORTUNITY**
>
> Visit a federal agency website and identify the types of programs, offices, or initiatives focused on rural health.

Section Review

In this section we have identified and discussed **federal agencies** as the second element comprising the support factor. Here are the four agencies funded to improve the health of rural populations: the Center for Disease control (CDC), the Office of Rural Health Policy (FORHP), the Rural Health Research Center Program, and the Office of Rural Mental Health Research. As we looked at each of these agencies, we briefly discussed that agency's role in improving health outcomes in rural areas. With the research, education, and interventions provided by these federal agencies, rural health issues such as suicide, black lung disease, and mental health needs are being tackled.

RUNNING CASE

Ms. Jones's Health Science Class

At one of the Ms. Jones's advisory meetings, several members suggested she explore the "payback options available to students." One member talked about how programs through the state Office of Rural Health were set up to help medical students pay education loans in exchange for working in underserved areas. Another member discussed how few local students knew about the National Health Science Corps. Advisory members decided that a good project for Ms. Jones's students would be exploring the various local, state, and national payback and assistance programs for students looking toward health care careers in rural areas.

LEARNING ASSESSMENT—FEDERAL AGENCIES

Take this learning assessment and then compare your responses to the answers provided at the end of the book. You may find there are elements of the support factor you would like to review to gain a better understanding

1. List the four federal agencies discussed in this section.
2. Provide some examples of rural health issues that the CDC has reported on.
3. Name FORHP's four main programs designed to increase health care access for rural populations.
4. The Rural Health Research Center Program is funded by the federal government to produce policy-relevant research on _____ _____ and _____ _____ in rural areas.
5. What is the ORMHR mandated to do by Congress?

National Programs/Organizations as an Element of the Support Factor

Because of the complexity of rural health, national organizations and programs supplement the work that is done by federal agencies. Some organizations can have funding priorities that support rural health care delivery (Kate B. Reynolds), track rural health statistics (Pew Foundation), or provide information and/or services to rural communities. We build on our knowledge of the federal agencies element, as we now focus on the national programs/organizations element and its impact on health care access in rural areas. We will focus on three national programs, which are Area Health Education Centers and County Health Rankings published by

Wisconsin Population Health Institute and the Cooperative Extension Service. We will focus on one national organization, the National Rural Health Association. The application opportunities at the end of the chapter leads to explore additional organizations devoted to rural health.

AREA HEALTH EDUCATION CENTERS

According to historical documents, Area Health Education Centers (AHECs) were created in 1971 by a federal law entitled the Comprehensive Health Manpower Training Act. The **AHEC** program was developed by Congress to recruit, train, and retain a health professions workforce committed to underserved populations (National AHEC

> **AHEC** is a public or nonprofit private organization that has a cooperative agreement or contract in effect with an entity that has received an award from HRSA under PHS Act Section 751(a) (1) or Section 751(a) (2). Such organizations may include hospitals, health organizations with accredited primary care training programs, accredited physician assistant educational programs associated with a college or university, and universities or colleges not operating a school of medicine or osteopathic medicine (National AHEC Organization, AHEC Directory, n.d.).

Organization, Mission and History, n.d.). Initially, 11 AHECs were funded. In 1976, Congress enacted the Health Professions Educational Assistance Act that helped focus the scope and programs offered by **AHECs** (Gessert & Smith, 1981).

The **AHEC** National Association website indicates that almost every state has at least one **AHEC**. In the United States and District of Columbia there are 46 **AHEC** programs with more than 261 centers (National AHEC Organization, n. d.). These centers share common missions and programs and engage in workforce development. Pipeline programs in which rural students learn about and engage in health career training programs serve to both encourage rural students to pursue health careers and to retain rural students in rural areas. According to the national **AHEC** website, thousands of students participate in pipeline programs that help students explore the variety of health professions open to them.

When feasible, **AHECs** offer student housing to those in health professions while on rural rotations. A new program in partnership with HRSA is the **AHEC** Scholars program in which interprofessional students attend didactic sessions and then complete clinical rotations in a variety of rural settings. These programs are created to both educate students about rural practice and recruit students upon graduation.

AHECs also provide support to existing rural practices in the form of practice management services. That is, **AHECs** may offer educational and consultation services for practitioners in areas such as streamlining billing or implementing new billing systems, establishing an outpatient quality assurance/improvement program, implementing patient-centered home models or group visits, or maximizing resources. Services in practice management help rural offices become more efficient, state-of-the-art settings that are responsive to the changes in health care processes.

A significant activity within **AHECs** is the continuing education programs offered to a variety of professionals. Educational programs might focus on recertification coursework, new updates in treatments and standards of care, or emerging issues such as COVID-19 or opioid addiction. Educational programs might focus on working with interpreters or training for health coaches. In short, these educational programs serve as an education bridge between new ideas in care and rural practitioners, who might find accessing such information problematic or applicable to their settings.

COUNTY HEALTH RANKINGS

Published yearly, the County Health Ranking and Roadmap initiative is a joint effort between University of Wisconsin Population Health Institute and the Robert Wood Johnson Foundation (County Health Rankings & Roadmaps, 2020). The rankings compare counties by reliably measuring data elements that impact health. Data elements include health behaviors, clinical care, social-economic items, and physical environment. Each item has a score and that county's score can be compared to another county within the state or to the state as a whole (County Health Rankings & Roadmaps). Comparisons can also be made with peer counties. Based on initial information or comparative information, local entities are able to identify key areas in which they wish to focus. For instance, the county may wish to implement programs to reduce alcohol-impaired driving deaths, to promote greater smoking cessation, to reduce preventable hospital stays, or to address severe housing issues. By reviewing data yearly, ongoing data collection can help program planners determine how effective interventions have been in meeting health goals. One caveat, however, is that data elements may change over time and the weight afforded each element in determining overall county ranking may also change. Thus, careful analysis of the information is necessary in order to completely understand health trends over time and to compare health elements with other elements.

COOPERATIVE EXTENSION SERVICE

The Cooperative Extension Service (CES) originated through a series of acts that designated federal funds paired with state-designated **land-grants universities**. The Smith-Lever Act of 1914 formed the Cooperative Extension Service and agricultural research stations to work in partnership with these **land-grant universities** for the purpose of enhancing agricultural and technical education.

Through a joint funding effort of states and the United States Department of Agriculture (USDA) most counties plus Tribal Nations have a Cooperative Extension Agent (USDA—National Institute of Food and Agriculture, n.d.). The Agents are integral to counties, particularly as rural community educators. Oftentimes the CES Agent lives in the county they serve and are some of the community voices discussed in regards to the sociocultural factor in Chapter 4. The Agent is tasked with translating agricultural research and science in a way that farmers and county residents can understand and find applications that are valuable to them. Agents work directly with farmers, agribusinesses, and communities to apply agriculture and food research.

CES provides nutrition programs such as the SNAP-Ed program (Supplemental Nutrition Assistance–Education). They partner locally with schools, churches, housing communities, nonprofits and employers to improve food choices. Youth development is also a focus of CES, with the best known program being 4-H programs. Serving ages 5–18, 4-H follows a curriculum that teaches leadership, civic engagement, science, and health (4-H Programs at a Glance, n.d.).

> **APPLICATION OPPORTUNITY**
>
> Go the County Health Ranking website (https://www.countyhealthrankings.org/). Choose two counties within your state, and compare overall rankings and item rankings. Determine which health item you would select to improve and the impact that changing that ranking would have on the overall health ranking in the county.

> The Association of Public and **Land-Grant Universities** defines a land-grant college or university as follows: "A **land-grant college or university** is an institution that has been designated by its state legislature or Congress to receive the benefits of the Morrill Acts of 1862, 1890, and 1994" (Association of Public & Land Grant Universities, n.d.).

NATIONAL ORGANIZATIONS

In addition to rural health focused national programs, there are professional and practitioner organizations devoted to rural health. One such organization is the National Rural Health Association. As its website states, "The National Rural Health Association (NRHA) is a national nonprofit membership organization with more than 21,000 members. ..." (2020).

The association's mission is to provide leadership on rural health issues through advocacy, communications, education, and research. The NRHA has a variety of programs. They are an advocacy group that gives presentations before Congress, federal agencies, the White

APPLICATION OPPORTUNITY

Visit the National Rural Health Association website:
https://www.ruralhealthweb.org/programs/
state-rural-health-associations
Find your state's rural health association listed
there. Then visit the state association to determine
the type of programs and services provided.

APPLICATION OPPORTUNITY

Conduct an internet search to identify at least three
foundations that fund rural health initiatives. As
a starting point, you may wish to review funders
listed on Rural Health Affairs website: https://www
.healthaffairs.org/doi/full/10.1377/hlthaff.2017.1220

House, and other policy makers. The NRHA have diverse programs that look at broad rural health issues (health disparity or rural emergency preparedness), as well as more focused concerns such as rural veteran's health or rural oral health. The NRHA delivers these programs through a variety of distribution channels: conferences, papers and publications including the *Rural Horizons* magazine and *Rural Health Voices* blog and their peer-reviewed journal *The Journal of Rural Health* that focuses on publishing advancing professional practice, research, and theory related to rural health.

Each state has a corresponding local rural health association. For instance, the NC Rural Health Leadership Alliance (Foundation for Health, 2020) serves as the statewide counterpart to the National Rural Health Association, as does the Rural Health Association of Tennessee (2020), which serves citizens of Tennessee. These state organizations help to distribute national news, concerns, and programs to the local rural health leaders, as well as bring forth local issues to a national focus.

While some associations may have broad rural health foci, some concentrate on key rural health issues or settings. For instance, The National Association of Rural Health Clinics (NARHC) focuses on clinics in rural areas and serves as an advocacy group on their behalf (2018). Still other national associations have historically provided financial assistance to rural health improvements, funds like the Commonwealth Fund (2020) or Kate B. Reynolds Charitable Trust in North Carolina. As rural health gains greater awareness, it is hoped that other associations and programs will emerge with a primary rural health focus.

Section Review

In this section we have looked at national programs/organizations as the third element comprising the support factor. We learned several strategies that AHEC uses to recruit, train, and retain health professional to care for underserved populations. Next, we explored the county-level comparative data categories the County Health Ranking and Roads Maps provides for guiding health care decision-making. Then found that the USDA helps fund and promote the Cooperative Extension Service and their partnerships with land-grant universities to produce application research important to agricultural populations. This section ends by introducing us to some of the national organizations that focus on rural health.

RUNNING CASE

Mrs. Jones's Health Science Class

The advisory meeting today was particularly insightful. Advisory members discussed how nontraditional careers were often overlooked when students thought about health careers. For instance, the computer science teacher mentioned that few students thought about health informatics as a possible career choice. This led to a recommendation that students in Ms. Jones's class complete a matrix of all career codes in the Bureau of Labor Statistics database that might have something to do with health and might offer broader options for students who do not want to enter a clinical career.

LEARNING ASSESSMENT—NATIONAL PROGRAMS/ORGANIZATIONS

Take this learning assessment and then compare your responses to the answers provided at the end of the book. You may find there are elements of the support factor you would like to review to gain a better understanding

1. List national organizations/programs discussed in this section.
2. Name one service offered or a purpose for each of the organizations/programs listed.
3. AHEC is a private, or for-profit, organization.
   a. True
   b. False
4. How often does County Health Rankings report data? Select the correct answer.
   a. Every 5 years
   b. Biannually
   c. Annually
   d. Every 2 years
5. What is the name of the act that formed the CES and agricultural research stations?

Telehealth as an Element of the Support Factor

In this section, we will explore the support factor element, telehealth. By now, you clearly understand the impact that distance from provider, health professional scarcities, and lack of integrated health care have on patients and clients in rural areas. The more remote, the greater the impact. One way to overcome the problem of remote access is through greater use of technology. We will explore three types of telehealth: telemedicine, telepsychiatry, and telepharmacy.

TELEMEDICINE

The terms telehealth and telemedicine are often used interchangeably. For our purposes, we will divide the two and consider the more narrow definition of telemedicine to be the use of technology to deliver medical care at a distance (HealthIT.gov, 2019), that is, a clinician delivering care to a patient at a distant location. The purpose of the technology is to provide or enhance medical care. Alternatively, telehealth "refers broadly to electronic and telecommunications technologies and services used to provide care and services at-a-distance ... including both clinical and non-clinical services" (American Academy of Family Practitioners, n.d.).

Teleconsultation typically involves establishing a communication link between doctors who request consultations on patients under their care and experts located in distant medical centers.

Telemedicine uses a broad range of technologies. Some, like videoconferencing, can occur in real time as when a physician examines a patient in a patient's home or in another setting like a nursing home or a prison. Sometimes this activity is called a televisit or a telepatient encounter. Alternatively, patient visits can be captured using a videoconference platform and then transmitted to another (sometimes a specialist). This asynchronous telemedicine episode does not require real-time patient interactions (Health Resources & Services Administration, 2019).

Telemedicine might also include technologies that aid in remote patient monitoring. One example is an asthma app that monitors asthma symptoms and sends data directly into the patient's chart (Digitalhealth, n.d.). Likewise, mobile data devices enable the home-health nurse visiting a patient to transmit data directly to a triage nurse or patient record. Devices help monitor patient conditions, record data in charts or patient records, and alert patients and providers of needed changes help to improve care, especially in remote or underserved areas.

Equally important is the ability of multiple health providers to input and access shared electronic data bases, including health records. This is aided by the Office of the National Coordinator for Health Information Technology (ONC), which is tasked with promoting a nationwide health information exchange to improve health care. Providers access shared electronic medical records and shared health records to help integrate care, reduce health costs by eliminating duplicative tests, reduce safety risks, and reduce medical errors. For example, a shared record enables multiple providers and specialists to have more comprehensive diagnostic information and better understand how their treatment plans fit into the treatment plans of others (HealthIT.gov, 2017).

Lastly, **telemedicine** also allows patients greater access and involvement in their care. Patients can view their charts in real time to query providers through secured portals and to input data into their own records. This expands the concept of patient partnership and increases the trust, transparency, and involvement of patients who lack access due to burdens of transportation, lost wages, or unavailable providers.

TELEPYSCHIATRY

As we have noted in previous chapters, mental health is particularly problematic in rural areas. First, there is a shortage of mental health professionals in rural areas. Professional shortages mean that patients might not be able to see a mental health specialist without having to travel long distances or that non-mental health providers take on the role, often with little or no specialty support (East Carolina University, 2020). Secondly, rural residents' health beliefs might dismiss the presence of mental health concerns. Lastly, health insurance of

---

> **APPLICATION OPPORTUNITY**
>
> Go to https://health.usnews.com/conditions/articles/innovative-telehealth-programs-across-medical-specialties, and identify other examples of **telemedicine** activities or programs.

> **APPLICATION OPPORTUNITY**
>
> Report on how different states/locations have implemented telemedicine in their rural areas. For instance, you might want to visit the New Mexico model: https://hsc.unm.edu/health/for-medical-professionals/access/about-telemedicine/ Or the University of Arizona model: https://telemedicine.arizona.edu/about-us/background/ Be sure to review the goals beyond direct patient care for these **telemedicine** programs.

> **Telepsychiatry** is the use of two-way real-time interactive audio and video between places of lesser and greater psychiatric expertise to provide and support psychiatric care when distance separates participants who are in different geographical locations (NC Division of Medical Assistance, 2018).

---

rural residents might only provide limited coverage for ongoing mental health visits. **Telepsychiatry** presents an option of providing specialty consultation and patient visits to rural populations. Fortunately, growing research tells us that **telepsychiatry** might serve to offset workforce shortages and deliver needed support and care, especially to heretofore underserved populations. Let us explore one such **telepsychiatry** program.

Since the mid-1990s, The Brody School of Medicine at East Carolina University has been providing **telepsychiatry** services, although telepsychiatry can trace its beginning to the 1950s (American Psychiatrist Association). Today, the East Carolina University Center for **Telepsychiatry** and E-Behavioral Health (CTeBH) is home to the North Carolina Statewide **telepsychiatry** program (NC-STeP). "The vision of NC-STeP is to assure that if an individual experiencing an acute behavioral health crisis enters an emergency department of a hospital anywhere in the state of North Carolina, s/he receives timely specialized psychiatric treatment through this program" (East Carolina University, n.d.). Currently, more than 80 hospital emergency rooms are enrolled in the telepsychiatry service. Similar to other telemedicine programs, the goal of this and other **telepsychiatry** services is to improve care (e.g., reduce unnecessary hospital admissions) and provide expert support, especially in rural areas.

TELEPHARMACY

In the telehealth element, we have thus far discussed telemedicine and, as an example of a specialty telemedical application, **telepsychiatry**. In this section, we want to look at **telepharmacy** as a newcomer to the telehealth care technology landscape and an example of the breadth that these technologies might cover. In its broadest definition, **telepharmacy** "is considered to be a way of delivering pharmaceutical products and care by the means of telecommunication to different patients" (eVisit).

Telepharmacy can take various forms. Community pharmacists through **telepharmacy** might serve to back up inpatient hospital pharmacists by way of remote order-entry review. A second model is the placement of a certified pharmacy technician supervised from afar by a pharmacist. A specialized example of **telepharmacy** may be the IV admixture route where technicians mix up IV-admixture but are supervised and reviewed from outside the clean area, thus saving time for the pharmacist to suit up and enter the clean room (ASHP, 2016, p. 3). **Telepharmacy** may enable pharmacists to engage in remote counseling with patients as they provide valuable information, education, and counseling for their clients (ASHP Statement on Telepharmacy, 2016).

Lastly, **telepharmacy** might include direct patient care services, including medication therapy management, especially for chronic disease, in which some states have authorized pharmacists under physician supervision to prescribe or adjust medication doses (National/Alliance of State Pharmacy Associations, 2018).

APPLICATION OPPORTUNITY

Find an example of **telepharmacy**, for instance North Dakota Telepharmacy Project: https://www.ndsu.edu/telepharmacy/how_telepharmacy_works/.

Section Review

In this section we have looked at **telehealth** as the fourth element making up the support factor. We discussed these three types of telehealth: **telemedicine**, **telepsychiatry**, and **telepharmacy**. We learned how telehealth can improve health care access by overcoming distance from providers, health professional shortages, and integration of health care for rural populations. We see that technology as way to overcome the remoteness of rural areas. As a closing thought, high-speed internet accessibility in every rural area does not exist. There is much to be done to deliver broadband to remote rural areas and to the homes of rural people.

RUNNING CASE

Mrs. Jones's Health Science Class

It has been helpful to have community members on the advisory group. The local physician mentioned that few students were aware of the impact that foreign medical and clinical personnel have on rural areas. This prompted Mr. Darvin, the government teacher, to say that he would introduce a module on rural health when he discusses contemporary immigration issues in his class. Community members offered to serve on a panel that looked at the contribution made by foreign-trained clinicians.

LEARNING ASSESSMENT—TELEHEALTH

Take this learning assessment and then compare your responses to the answers provided at the end of the book. You may find there are elements of the support factor you would like to review to gain a better understanding

1. List three types of telehealth discussed in this section.
2. Telehealth can help minimize the impact that a patient's distance from their provider has on access to care.
   a. True
   b. False
3. Telehealth has no impact on health professional scarcities and the lack of integrated health care for patients and clients in rural areas.
   a. True
   b. False
4. Name two technologies that telemedicine utilizes.
5. The Brody School of Medicine at _____ _____ University Center for telepsychiatry and E-Behavioral Health (CTeBH) is home to the North Carolina Statewide telepsychiatry program (NC-STeP).

Rural Health Interventions as an Element of the Support Factor

In this final section of the chapter, we turn our attention to the rural health intervention element within the support factor. We will explore two initiatives that have been undertaken to provide support to rural residents with the aim of improving rural health. The first, health centers, is an infrastructure example of how an intervention addresses the access issue. The other, expanded roles, is an example of how changing practice guidelines/roles can leverage workforce resources in traditionally underserved areas. There are many more initiatives, but these examples serve to exemplify the work that is being done to help provide support to rural communities and improve rural health.

HEALTH CENTERS

As discussed throughout the chapters, access to care includes the presence in the community of highly qualified and affordable care options. To provide a resource to underserved areas, the federal government (HRSA) funded a network of health centers to provide primary and preventive care under Section 330 of the Public Health Service Act (https://uscode.house .gov/view.xhtml?edition=prelim&req=42+usc+254b&f+treesort&fq+true&num=2-&hl=true). In addition to federal funding, these Federally Qualified Health Centers (FQHC) may be community health centers, migrant health centers, health care for the homeless, or health centers for residents of public housing (Health Resources & Services Administration, May, 2018), These centers qualify for special reimbursement from Medicare and Medicaid (FQHC. org). Some local health centers may not be eligible for federal funding but are still eligible for the Medicare and Medicaid enhancement payments—these centers are referred to as *look-alikes*. Both Federally Qualified Health Centers and look-alikes provide comprehensive primary health care services and must meet all Health Center program requirements (Health Resources & Services Administration November,2018). The requirements include setting fees based on a sliding payment scale, being governed by a board that includes patients, providing care that includes dental and mental health services, and most importantly, serving underserved areas (FQHC.org). Currently one in five rural residents receives care through a FQHC or look-alike (Health Resources and Services Administration, Health Center Program).

According to the HRSA website (2018), "... all health centers, including look-alikes, gain access to

> **Federally Qualified Health Centers** are community-based health care providers that receive funds from HRSA.

- Federally Qualified Health Center Prospective Payment System reimbursement for services to Medicare (https://www.cms.gov/medicare/medicare-fee-for-service-payment/fqhcpps) and Medicaid (https://www.medicaid.gov) beneficiaries;
- 340B Drug Pricing Program (https://www.hrsa.gov/opa), discounts for pharmaceutical products;
- Free vaccines for uninsured and underinsured children through the Vaccines for Children Program; (https://www.cdc.gov/vaccines/programs/vfc/index.html); and
- Assistance in the recruitment and retention of primary care providers through the National Health Service Corps (https://nhsc.hrsa.gov)."

Contrary to many beliefs, Federally Qualified Health Centers are not rundown buildings with lesser programs or staff. There is strong evidence that these health centers increase access and reduce negative outcomes, while providing quality and affordable care (County Health Rankings & Roadmaps, 2016). In many rural areas, health centers are the medical home for much of the population. Equally important, many of the centers' patients are from underrepresented populations, making centers one of the most effective health delivery venues for reducing racial and ethnic health disparities (Community Health Connection, n.d.).

> **APPLICATION OPPORTUNITY**
>
> Identify a Federally Qualified Health Center in your area. Describe the type of services provided, the staff that provides such services, and the number of patients seen each year. If possible, take a live or virtual tour of the facility.

EXPANDED ROLES

The lack of health and health care resources in a community is a critical component of poorer health outcomes for rural residents. In an effort to augment these scarce resources, new health roles have emerged. These roles leverage the knowledge and skills of persons who are familiar with the community and are in place there and address critical needs of rural patients. We will look at four roles: community health worker, health coach, patient navigator, and community paramedics. While these roles may overlap, each contributes unique services to the citizens in rural areas.

> **Community Health Worker:** A frontline public health worker who is a trusted member of and/or has an unusually close understanding of the community served (American Public Health Association, n.d.).

Community Health Worker

Persons knowledgeable about the community have much to offer the health and health care system. Often trusted by fellow residents, **community health workers** can help implement organizations and medical personnel programs in the community, enhance acceptance of health initiatives, and serve as advocates for the needs of the community (American Public Health Association, n.d.). In some communities, **community health workers** may assist patients/clients in connecting with needed community resources or help provide basic care (e.g., blood pressure screening) for select patients. The importance of **community health care workers** connecting patients to services, especially in resource-poor areas, cannot be underestimated in the goal of reducing poor health outcomes in these areas.

Health Coach

Another expanded role that has found a natural home in rural areas is **health coach**. By most definitions, **health coaches** work with patients to help empower patients to adopt and sustain healthy lifestyles to improve health outcomes. For instance, **health coaches** might help patients who have diabetes change their eating or physical activity lifestyles as a means of better controlling their diabetes. These behavioral changes are intended to positively improve health outcomes. By coaching patients, **health coaches** seek to improve self-management and empowerment (Health Coach Institute, 2021).

Health Coach: The National Society of Health Coaches describes evidence-based health coaching (EBHC) as the use of evidence-based skillful conversation, clinical strategies, and interventions to actively and safely engage clients in health behavior change to better self-manage their health, health risk, and acute and chronic conditions, resulting in optimal wellness, lowered health risk, improved health outcomes, and decreased health costs (n.d.).

APPLICATION OPPORTUNITY

Look at various certification programs for **health coaches** or patient navigators, and identify who is offering such programs and how someone can obtain a certification.

Patient Navigator: "According to the American Medical Association (AMA), a **patient navigator** is someone whose primary responsibility is to provide personalized guidance to patients as they move through the healthcare system" (Patient Engagement Hit, 2018).

Patient Navigator

A third role that has a function in rural health improvement is that of **patient navigator**. Gaining prominence in the 1990 and then achieving significant support in the Affordable Care Act, a patient navigator helps patients understand and navigate the health care system. **Patient navigators** are often called to help patients understand and complete insurance forms, as well as describing what is covered. As we have seen in previous chapters, patients who do not have a lot of contact with the system, who may not have the expertise (or the time) to understand the nuances of the health care system, and who often must utilize multiple components of the system (care, rehabilitation, therapies, diagnostics) can become so frustrated with the system that they give up or miss available resources. The patient navigator is there to ensure that appropriate patient resources are understood, maximized, and utilized.

APPLICATION OPPORTUNITY

For a more comprehensive list of community paramedics tasks see the following website: https://www.ncsl.org/research/health/expanding-the-primary-care-role-of-first-responder.aspx#CP.

Community Paramedics

Perhaps a newer concept/role in some areas is the role of **community paramedics**. The idea is to utilize the expertise of existing emergency medical technicians and paramedics that currently are employed and reside in the community. These individuals already know the health care system, have systems in place to provide care in the community, and have the trust of community residents. **Community paramedics** may be asked to assess nonemergency chronic care patients, to give immunizations, and to follow homebound patients, just to name a few of the proposed tasks that can be undertaken. The creation of a **community paramedic** program may also have financial benefits: fewer nonemergency transports or calls, greater utilization of existing resources, and services to patients that reduce hospitalizations and enhance at-home care.

Section Review

In this section we have looked at **health interventions** as the fifth and last element making up the support factor. We discussed two examples of rural health interventions: rural health centers and expanded roles. The initiatives we explored provide support to rural residents with the aim of improving rural health. The first, health centers, is an infrastructure example of how an intervention addresses access issues. The second, expanded roles, provided an example of how changing practice guidelines/roles can leverage workforce resources in traditionally underserved areas.

LEARNING ASSESSMENT—HEALTH INTERVENTIONS

Take this learning assessment and then compare your responses to the answers provided at the end of the book. You may find there are elements of the support factor you would like to review to gain a better understanding

1. What are the two examples of rural health interventions discussed in this section?
2. Which of these two examples provides an infrastructure intervention addressing the issue of health care access?
3. Which of the two examples of rural health interventions involves changing practice guidelines/roles to leverage workforce resources in traditionally underserved areas?
4. Federally Qualified Health Centers (FQHC) includes _____ _____ health care providers that receive funds from HRSA.
5. List the four expanded health care roles discussed in this section.

CHAPTER SUMMARY

In this chapter we explored the fifth factor of the Rural Health Framework: The support factor. We discovered that support comes in several forms: financial support, programmatic, legislative, or regulatory. Additionally, we saw that support may also come from agencies or groups whose mission it is to inform policy makers, influencers, or investors. We examined how support comes from local, state, or national entities and may focus on a population or geographical area. In this chapter we will delved into five elements that make up the support factor: local governance, federal agencies, national programs/organizations, telehealth, and health interventions.

Chapter 6 gave us a different perspective than the previous chapters. Rather than looking at comparisons between urban and rural or the manifestation of health outcomes, we began with the premise that rural areas require special attention because of poor health outcomes and ongoing needs. Thus, this chapter did not compare the support vehicles between urban and rural, but instead explored those specific support elements that are found in rural areas and focused on rural health concerns.

To capture all the support elements, fill in the Support Factor County Assessment Grid Template (see Table 6.1). By answering each of the questions on the grid, no element is excluded or minimized. Instead, the completed grid allows us to efficiently view key characteristics that are known to impact the health of the citizens of that county.

Not only can we use the grid to provide a snapshot of the support elements in the county, but we can use the grid to help us explain what we are viewing and even to identify missing issues that might help inform us as to the nature of rural health needs. To practice applying the Support Factor County Assessment Grid Template address the two learner challenges at the end of this chapter.

These factors and elements do not stand alone in their impact on rural health. In previous chapters we examined the impact of the geographical factor and the economical factor, the demographical factor, and the sociocultural factor. Now as we complete our understanding of the support factor on rural health, we conclude the journey of identifying issues that impact rural health. In the next and final chapter you will have the opportunity to apply all the data/facts you have compiled to address a rural health case assessment.

TABLE 6.1   Support Factor County Assessment Grid Template

Factor	Elements	County Data	Source & Comments
Support	Local Governance	Local boards of health	List the names of the members of the BOH. Compile their contact information.
		County commissioners	List the names of the county commissioners. Compile their contact information.
	Federal Agencies	Centers for Disease Control (CDC)	Compile information about any health interventions currently in progress or planned that may impact the county.
		Office of Rural Health	
		Policy (FORHP)	Compile information regarding funds available for the special populations within the county.
		Rural Health Research Center Program	
		Office of Rural Mental Health Research (ORMHR)	
	National Programs/Organizations	AHECs	Explore these programs/organizations for initiatives, data, or model interventions that have would benefit the county.
		County Health Rankings	
		CES	
		National Organizations	

TABLE 6.1   Support Factor County Assessment Grid Template *(continued)*

Factor	Elements	County Data	Source & Comments
	Telehealth	Telemedicine Telepsychiatry Telepharmacy	Find out if any or all are available to residents in the county.
	Health Interventions	Health centers (FQHC, look-alikes, or others)	Locate the health centers accessible to residents in the county. Compile facts about services.
		Expanded roles (community health workers, health coaches, patient navigators)	Identify if the county residents have access to any health providers in these expanded roles. Compile contact information and services offered.

CHAPTER ACTIVITY—LEARNING CHALLENGE

Below are two learning challenges designed to help apply the support factor's elements in a systematic review. The learning challenge can be completed individually or in small groups.

Learning Challenge 1: Using your county or a selected county, complete the Support Factor Assessment Grid. Be sure to populate each element with comprehensive data elements, and be sure to include all sources from which data/facts were obtained.

Learning Challenge 2: The Health Interventions portion of your grid is complete. Are there any additional data/facts you have learned about that the grid did not include? Consider the data/facts you have collected, and add any *additional information* that you may have identified about your county.

CHAPTER ACTIVITY—PRACTICE VIGNETTES

Vignette 1: The local AHEC has asked you to help them identify new topics of interest to practitioners in your area. They wish the session(s) to be interprofessional as well as relevant to the needs of practitioners. As a starting point, they have asked that you help them think through the following planning issues:

a. How would you go about identifying the practitioners in your area that AHEC should survey to assess needs and interests?

b. Who in your area has an established interest in workforce development that might help to cosponsor an event (either financially or with publicity support)?

c. Where might AHEC planners look to see existing information about workforce needs in your area?

Vignette 2: The board of health is reviewing the newly released County Health Rankings. While some areas have improved, others have not. Of concern is the increase in alcohol-related issues (excessive drinking, alcohol impaired driving deaths). In trying to determine what to do next, they want your help. Specifically, they are interested in the following:

a. Ideas for organizations or associations that might address specific health concerns related to alcohol or substance abuse issues.
b. How might rural agencies, such as the Agriculture Extension Service, partner with prevention programs?
c. Who in the county might be a partner in helping to reverse this trend line?

Vignette 3: The county commissioners are reviewing a recommendation from the board of health and Concerned Citizens for Health to create more walking trails in the county. They are interested in finding knowledgeable resources to help them in their deliberations. They have asked you to

a. Identify federal agencies that might have data the county commissions might find informative.
b. List state or county agencies have data that might be similarly useful.
c. Describe why having more open spaces (including walking trails) are an important rural health intervention.

REFERENCES—LOCAL GOVERNANCE

AccessKent Kent County Michigan. (n.d.). Health department. https://www.accesskent.com/Health/

Byers, Jacqueline J. (2008, November). Research brief—what do county commissioners do all day? https://www.naco.org/sites/default/files/documents/What%20Do%20County%20Commissioners%20Do%20All%20Day.pdf

Iowa Department of Public Health. (2018). Local board of health. https://idph.iowa.gov/Portals/1/userfiles/147/BOH%20Brochure%20%2001-03-18.pdf

Massachusetts Association of Health Boards. (n.d.). Boards of health. https://www.mahb.org/boards-of-health

Tri-County Health Department. (n.d.). Board of health. https://www.tchd.org/438/Board-of-Health.

REFERENCES—FEDERAL AGENCIES

Health Resources & Services Administration. (2019, August). Rural health policy. https://www.hrsa.gov/rural-health/policy/index.html

Health Resources & Services Administration. (2020, July). Telehealth programs. https://www.hrsa.gov/rural-health/telehealth

National Institute of Mental Health. (n.d.). Office of Rural Mental Health Research. https://www.nimh.nih.gov/about/organization/od/office-of-rural-mental-health-research-ormhr.shtml

National Institute of Mental Health. (2018, May 30). Mental health and rural America: Challenges and opportunities. https://www.nimh.nih.gov/news/media/2018/mental-health-and-rural-america-challenges-and-opportunities.shtml

REFERENCES—NATIONAL PROGRAMS/ORGANIZATIONS

4-H Programs at a Glance. (n.d.). Types of 4-H programs. https://4-h.org/parents/programs-at-a-glance/.

Association of Public & Land-Grant Universities. (n.d.). Land-grant university FAQ. https://www.aplu.org/about-us/history-of-aplu/what-is-a-land-grant-university/

Clark, J. K., Bean, M., Raja, S., Loveridge, S., Freedgood, J., & Hodgson, K. (2017). Cooperative extension and food system change: Goals, strategies and resources. *Agriculture and Human Values, 34*(2), 301–316. doi:http://dx.doi.org/10.1007/s10460-016-9715-2

The Commonwealth Fund. (2020). Foundation history. https://www.commonwealthfund.org/about-us/foundation-history

County Health Rankings & Roadmaps. (2020). About us. https://www.countyhealthrankings.org/about-us

County Health Rankings & Roadmaps. (2020). 2020 County Health Rankings state reports. https://www.countyhealthrankings.org/

Foundation for Health. (2020). NC Rural Health Leadership Alliance. https://foundationhli.org/programs/nc-rural-health-leadership-alliance/

Gessert, Charles E. & Smith, D. (1981). The National AHEC program: Review of its progress and considerations for the 1980s. *Public Health Reports (1974-), 96*(2), 116–120. http://www.jstor.org/stable/4596459.

Kaufman, A., Boren, J., Koukel, S., Ronquillo, F., Davies, C., & Nkouaga, C. (2017). Agriculture and health sectors collaborate in addressing population health. *Annals of Family Medicine, 15*(5), 475–480. doi:10.1370/afm.2087

National AHEC Organization. (n.d.). AHEC directory. https://www.nationalahec.org/index.php/about-us/ahec-directory

National AHEC Organization. (n.d.). Mission and history. https://www.nationalahec.org/ page/MissionHistoryBoard

National Association of Rural Health Clinics. About us. (2018). https://www.web.narhc.org/ narhc/ESX_About_Us_2.asp

National Rural Health Association. (2020). About NRHA. https://www.ruralhealthweb.org/ about-nrha

Rural Health Association of Tennessee. (2020). Rural health matters. http://www.rhat.org/

United States Department of Agriculture—National Institute of Food and Agriculture. (n.d.). Extension. https://nifa.usda.gov/extension

REFERENCES—TELEHEALTH

American Academy of Family Practitioners. (n.d.). What's the difference between telemedicine and telehealth? https://www.aafp.org/media-center/kits/telemedicine-and-telehealth.html

American Psychiatric Association. (n.d.). History of telepsychiatry. https://www.psychiatry .org/psychiatrists/practice/telepsychiatry/toolkit/history-of-telepsychiatry

ASHP Statement on Telepharmacy. (2016). Prepress version [pdf]. https://www.ashp.org/-/ media/assets/pharmacy-informaticist/docs/sopit-bp-telepharmacy-statement.ashx

Digitalhealth. (n.d.). Asthma app monitors children's symptoms to reduce risk of attacks. https://www.digitalhealth.net/2019/08/asthma-app-childrens-symptoms-reduce-attacks/

East Carolina University. (n.d.). NC-STeP welcome. https://www.ecu.edu/cs-dhs/ncstep/

East Carolina University. (2020). Center for Telepsychiatry and e-Behavioral Health. https:// www.ecu.edu/cs-dhs/telepsychiatry/

eVisit. (n.d.). What is telepharmacy? https://evisit.com/resources/what-is-telepharmacy.

Health Resources & Services Administration. (2019). Telehealth programs. https://www.hrsa .gov/rural-health/telehealth/

HealthIT.gov. (2017). Improve care coordination. https://www.healthit.gov/topic/ health-it-basics/improve-care-coordination

HealthIT.gov. (2019). What is telehealth? How is telehealth different from telemedicine? https:// www.healthit.gov/faq/what-telehealth-how-telehealth-different-telemedicine

National Alliance of State Pharmacy Associations. (Nov. 9, 2018). Pharmacist prescribing: Statewide protocols and more. https://naspa.us/resource/swp/

NC Division of Medical Assistance. (January 1, 2018). Medicaid and Health Choice Clinical Coverage Policy No: 1H [pdf]. https://files.nc.gov/ncdma/documents/files/1-H.pdf

REFERENCES—HEALTH INTERVENTIONS

American Public Health Association. (n.d.). Community health workers. https://www.apha.org/apha-communities/member-sections/community-health-workers

Community Health Connection. (n.d.). Economic impact of CHC. https://communityhealthconnection.org/about-us/economic-impact-of-chc/

County Health Rankings & Roadmaps. (2016, November 15). Federally qualified health centers (FQHC). https://www.countyhealthrankings.org/take-action-to-improve-health/what-works-for-health/strategies/federally-qualified-health-centers-fqhcs

FQHC.org. (n.d.). What is an FQHC? https://www.fqhc.org/what-is-an-fqhc/ Health Resources & Services Administration (n.d.) HRSA Health Center Program. https://bphc.hrsa.gov/sites/default/files/bphc/about/healthcenterfactsheet.pdf

Health Resources & Services Administration. (2018, May). Federally qualified health centers. https://www.hrsa.gov/opa/eligibility-and-registration/health-centers/fqhc/index.html

Health Resources & Services Administration. (2018, November). Health center program look-alikes. https://bphc.hrsa.gov/programopportunities/lookalike/index.html

HRSA Health Center Program. (2018, November). What is a health center? https://bphc.hrsa.gov/about/what-is-a-health-center/index.html

The National Society of Health Coaches. (n.d.). NHSC frequently asked questions. https://www.nshcoa.com/faq#q31

Patient Engagement Hit. (2018, August 10). How non-clinical staff enable patient engagement, care coordination. https://patientengagementhit.com/features/how-non-clinical-staff-enable-patient-engagement-care-coordination

Figure Credit

IMG 6.1: Source: https://www.flickr.com/photos/usdagov/33019552526/.

Chapter Seven

Rural Health Case Assessments

Introduction

This last chapter provides application opportunities employing the Rural Health Framework by means of six case assessments. Before beginning the case assessments, look over the example county data grid and read on to see how the county specific data/facts are utilized in planning an early stoke prevention program. This example case assessment demonstrates how to operationalize the framework by compiling data/facts that are then used to inform rural health decision-making. The sources for county data/facts are published research, online databases, county organizations, and others. Further county data/facts can be gleaned by visiting the county and interviewing community leaders and residents of the county.

In the process of gathering county information, the need to seek additional data/facts not depicted within the framework sometimes arises. This further investigation is similar to a health care provider completing a patient's history physical form. In the process, the health care professional's findings and judgment spawns additional information gathering that refines the health interventions. One last consideration regarding compiling county data/facts: There are categories of data where county-to-county and county-to-state comparisons prove insightful when seeking to address rural health concerns.

Rural Health Case Assessment—Example

STROKE PREVENTION PROGRAM

You are asked by the Community Partners for Health and Wellness for input regarding a stroke prevention program that is a combination of health education and health resource infrastructure. In anticipation of a formal proposal request from the State Health Director, you are to conduct an assessment of Sampson County utilizing the Rural Health Framework (RHF). Then, based on county specific data/facts you compile:

1. Identify sub populations within the county that should be the priority for the stroke prevention program.
2. Identify health education and resource infrastructure currently available in the county, and suggest additional health education and resource infrastructure that is needed for a successful program.

RESPONSE TO THE COMMUNITY PARTNERS FOR HEALTH AND WELLNESS

Data from the Centers for Disease Control (CDC) reveals African Americans are most at risk for stroke, while the Latinos are experiencing a rise in stroke death rates. The CDC indicates the age group at risk for stroke is not just people 65 and older. Research has demonstrated that 34% of people hospitalized for stroke are less than 65. Other indicators for people at risk for stroke are HBP, high cholesterol, smoking, obesity, and diabetes (Centers for Disease Control and Prevention, 2020).

#1 Identify sub populations within Sampson County that should be priority.

The above CDC information about strokes is employed to identify populations within Sampson County that should be priority for the stroke prevention program. Sampson County's African American population is 26.6% and Latino population 20.6%. With a total population of 63,531, these two ethic groups represent 29,986 Sampson County residents. Looking at age to identify people at risk, there are 11,437 (18%) people who are older than 65 (County Health Rankings & Roadmaps, 2020). A recommendation for gathering more age-related data would be to examine Sampson Regional hospitalization records for patients (who reside in the county) admitted with pre-stroke symptoms or strokes. There are five FQHCs in the county that could also provide more age-specific data regarding persons at risk. The FQHCs are Goshen Medical Center, Tri-County Community Health Council Harrells, Tri-County Community Health Council Dunn, Tri-County Community Health Council Clinton, and Community Health Council (Coharie Tribe, 2020). This additional data could potentially identify a wider or more varied age ranges to be included.

#2 Identify health education and resource infrastructure currently available in the county, and describe additional health education and resource infrastructure that is needed for a successful program.

Two health initiatives are identified that would contribute to a stroke prevention program. The State of the County Health (SOTCH) report (2018) mentions a Sampson County Health Department and Sampson County Partners for Healthy Carolinians Task Force (SCPFHC) collaboration (Sampson County Health Department, n.d., SOTCH, 2018). Sampson Regional Medical Center's Journey to Health is an 8-week program focusing on changing basic behaviors to move toward a healthier lifestyle and away from obesity. Sampson County Health Department and partnering agencies promoted the 2018 Eat Smart, Move More—Maintain, Don't Gain! Holiday Challenge (SOTCH, 2018). These two programs could be enhanced to help address risk factors for stroke, which include high blood pressure, high cholesterol, smoking, obesity, and diabetes. Changes to these programs and any newly developed programs should keep in mind the two target populations, African Americans and Latinos.

Identifying major employers in the county provides insight into insurance coverage obtainable to county residents who may work for companies located within the county. The major employers are Smithfield Foods, Sampson County Schools, Prestage Farms, Hog Slat Company, County of Sampson, Sampson Regional Medical Center, Clinton City Schools, Walmart Associates, NC Dept. of Public Safety, and DI & B Enterprises (SOTCH, 2018). Having insurance increases access to health care, along with other benefits such as paid sick leave and paid time off. With those benefits, a person would not have to sacrifice wages to attend a health appointment or be fearful of losing their job for being absent from work. Special attention when planning a stroke prevention program should be given to those employed in small businesses or self-employed. People with these types of employment lack these benefits and may be denied or self-deny access to health care. Rural residents may depend on seasonal jobs or part-time jobs, further decreasing access to health interventions.

Public and private health care facilities, along with emergency services and health care providers should be considered in planning. In a rural area like Sampson County, the Farm Extension Service is often a partner in health programs. The Sampson County Health Department and Sampson County Regional Hospital are both located in the county seat of Clinton (North Carolina Cooperative Extension, 2020). Two clinics in the county that would be valuable resources for the stroke program are Clinton Medical Clinic—Primary Care and Sampson Medical Group. The Department of Social Services' main location is in Clinton. They currently have programs for adults in areas such as nutrition, which could augment an educational aspect of the stroke program. Primary Care Physicians per 10,000 population is 4.7, which is low compared to the state at 7 per 10,000 population (Sampson County, 2019, Community Health Needs Assessment). Increasing the number of primary care physicians would benefit the stroke prevention efforts in the county. Some providers do offer telehealth, which is covered by Medicaid, Medicare, and NCBCBS. Increasing telehealth access can help maximize health professionals' ability to reach more patients. Other levels of providers could be recruited to the area, such as nurse practitioners and health coaches who could work in the program. The County Extension Service (CES) is located in Clinton, and the director is Eileen Coitee (North Carolina Cooperative Extension, 2020). CES in rural areas provides health education and outreach, making this agency a potential partner for the stroke prevention program. Similarly, the Board of Health with Paul Bradshaw, as chairman would be essential in program planning (North Carolina's Sampson County, n.d.).

The stroke prevention program must consider the culture of the Sampson County people and culture's impact on health choices. Since our target populations are African Americans and Latinos, their health beliefs and values should be understood and incorporated when planning, as much as possible. There may be mistrust of health care providers and of conventional medicine. Family members and folk healers are viewed as trusted sources for remedies to health concerns. Social capital in rural areas is a support and information network comprised of friends, family, neighbors, church family, and coworkers. If these networks could be tapped into it would positively impact acceptance of the stroke program. There are gathering places such as hair salons and barber shops that are trusted places with familiar people who could promote the program and share information about stroke prevention. Likewise, faith-based organizations and faith leader are trusted in rural communities. These organizations also have established programs and volunteers that can become partners and should be part of program planning and implementation.

Festivals and community events held in Sampson County can be venues for the stroke prevention program. Health screenings and education can be offered at the festivals. Sampson County festivals and events include Sampson County Ag Day, Alive After Five concert series, Veterans Day Celebration, Hubb's Farm–Field of Dreams, Sampson County History Museum Day, Battle of the Butts Cook-off, Fall Festival, Halloween Hustle, and Rocking for the Arts (Sampson County History Museum, n.d.).

Location is a consideration when planning the stroke prevention, relative to increasing access and reaching the most people. The county seat of Clinton is fairly centrally located with Harrells being the population center that is most distant to the county seat, located in the eastern tip of the county. Then there is Newton Grove, population 600, in the western tip of county. Roseboro, population 1,267, is located near the southern border midway into the county. Autryville, population <500, is located near the southern border midway into the county. Turkey, population <500, is located near the northern border midway into the county. Spivey's Corner, population <500, is located near Newton Grove in the western portion of the county. Salemburg, population <500, is located further within the border, between Clinton and Autryville. Last, there is Garland, located just above Harrells, with a population of 808 people (Image 7.1) (Sampson County Map, 2004).

Another element that impacts health care access is the roads county residents travel to access health care. Clinton has four major roads intersecting at the county seat. They are numbered

701, 24, 421, and 403. Here are other population centers with their major roads: Turkey has 24, Harrells has 421, Garland has 701, Autryville has 24, Roseboro has 24, and Newton Grove has 13 (Image 7.1, Sampson County Map). When planning a stroke prevention program, consideration should be given to ease of travel to the health care site.

Sampson County has five bodies of water: Black River, South River, Six Run Creek, Great Coharie Creek, Little Coharie Creek and all its tributaries (Image 7.1 Sampson County Map). The county water features might be utilized as part of an exercise program to improve health behaviors and encourage physical activity. These rivers should also be considered in terms of their physical relationship to roads and whether travel may be negatively impacted during certain times of the year.

There are few obstacles to air flow in rural areas, allowing pollen, dust, agricultural gases and chemicals, and smoke to travel long distances. Confined animal feeding operations affect air quality, resulting in increased respiratory illnesses, migraines, and depression. Smoke from forest fires can cause worsening of respiratory conditions and heart conditions. Seasonal pollen produced from heavy vegetation in rural areas increases asthma symptoms. Sampson County has sources that generate each of these types of poor air quality conditions. A stroke prevention program that may involve outdoor activities or exercise should consider air quality in certain areas.

Sampson County lies in the coastal plains of North Carolina where the weather can be extreme at times. For example, hurricane season begins in late August extending into early November. Those who plan health initiatives should take into account weather patterns of the area. Outdoor activities should be planned when temperatures are more favorable to avoid adverse health events from hypothermia or hyperthermia.

This concludes our response to the Community Partners for Health and Wellness. The Rural Health Framework with Sampson County data follows this narrative and supplies all data and sources utilized to compose the county assessment.

TABLE 7.1 Sampson County, North Carolina County Assessment Utilizing the Rural Health Framework.

Factor	Element	County Data	Comments
		Geographical Factor	
	Location	County Map	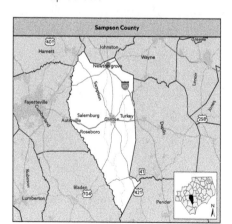
		Describe topology issues if not evident on map.	Coastal Plains of North Carolina—flatland, farmland, and forest. Second largest county in NC. Located 1 hour from Raleigh, the NC state capital.
		Surrounding counties	Johnston, Wayne, Duplin, Pender, Bladen, Cumberland, and Harnett Counties See map below:

TABLE 7.1   Sampson County, North Carolina County Assessment Utilizing the
Rural Health Framework *(continued)*.

Factor	Element	County Data	Comments
		Population Density Give the square miles in county and population per square mile.	67.1 people per square[1] Square miles 944.74 Total population 63,531[2]
		County Seat Name and locate the county seat. Describe how central or not central the county seat is relative to other population centers	Clinton Nearly centrally located. Harrells is a population center that is most distant to the county seat. More description about population centers follows below.
		Population Centers Give location of major population centers. Give population numbers for these centers	Newton Grove—population 600—in western tip of county—located within 45 miles of both Raleigh and Fayetteville. Roseboro—population 1,267—near the southern border midway the county—located close to Fayetteville Autryville—population <500—located near southern border midway the county. Turkey—population <500—located near northern border midway the county. Spivey's Corner—population <500—near Newton Grove in the western portion of the county. Salemburg—population <500—further within the border between Clinton and Autryville. Harrells—population <500—located in eastern tip of county Garland—population 808

1   Sampson County. (2019). Community Health Needs Assessment. https://cms4.revize.com/revize/sampsoncounty/document_center/Health/2019/2019%20Sampson_County%20CHNA%20Report%20FINAL.pdf

2   United States Census. (2018). QuickFacts Sampson County, North Carolina. https://www.census.gov/quickfacts/sampsoncountynorthcarolina

TABLE 7.1 Sampson County, North Carolina County Assessment Utilizing the Rural Health Framework *(continued)*.

Factor	Element	County Data	Comments
	Roads	Identify roads throughout the county, and describe these in terms for primary or secondary roads.	I40, I95, US HWY 701, US HWY 421, HWY 24, and US HWY 13.
		Identify any corridors of disease in the county.	I-95 major north–south corridor. I-40 major east–west corridor.
		Describe health statistics relative to roads. Vehicular accidents & fatalities.	18 fatalities in 2018 and 25 in 2016. The 2018 SOTCH lists MVA 7th in list of 10 leading causes of death. CHNA age-adjusted rate due to MVA 2012-2016 29.2 deaths/100,000 populations. Compared to NC 14.1/100,000 pop.[3] (Note: A comparison to counties in the region may be appropriate.)
		Placement of EMS and response time.	There are 16 Fire/EMS Stations located in the county with 13 of those stations located from Clinton west and the remaining 6 east of Clinton.[4] See map below:

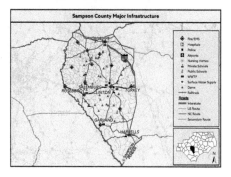

3   North Carolina 2018 Traffic Crash Facts. (n.d.) https://connect.ncdot.gov/business/DMV/CrashFactsDocuments/2018%20Crash%20Facts.pdf

4   Hurricane Matthew Resilient Redevelopment Plan. (May 2017). https://files.nc.gov/rebuildnc/documents/matthew/rebuildnc_sampson_plan_combined.pdf

TABLE 7.1 Sampson County, North Carolina County Assessment Utilizing the Rural Health Framework *(continued)*.

Factor	Element	County Data	Comments
	Air	Describe air quality. For instance: Particulate matter, CAFOs, organic, dust pollen	These are animal and plant sources that impact air quality:[5]
			Soybeans 67,379 acres
			Corn for grain 36,268 acres
			Vegetables 22,453 acres
			Forage 18,410 acres
			Wheat for grain 14,056 acres
			Meat chickens 5,969,281
			Laying chickens 313,878
			Pullets 318,338
			Turkeys 4,594,777
			Cattle 21,430
			Goats 939
			Swine 1,884,585
			Equine 820
			Sheep and lambs 216
			Additionally, forest and vegetation such as grasses and weeds should be considered.
		Describe air flow—are there many obstacles to impede air flow?	There are few obstacles such as tall buildings and other structures that create windbreaks. Average wind speed varies during the year 6.4 mph to 9.6 mph.
		List major air related health concerns in the county.	Respiratory illnesses and mental health concerns related to malodors from CAFOs. Chronic lower respiratory disease is the 5th leading cause of death under age 75.
	Water	Locate major bodies of water in the county and describe how used (drinking, transportation, recreation, commercial fishing, etc.).	Black River South River Six Run Creek Great Coharie Creek Little Coharie Creek and all tributaries

---

5   Census of Agriculture County Profile. (2017). Sampson County North Carolina. https://www.nass.usda.gov/Publications/AgCensus/2017/Online_Resources/County_Profiles/North_Carolina/cp37163.pdf

TABLE 7.1   Sampson County, North Carolina County Assessment Utilizing the
Rural Health Framework *(continued)*.

Factor	Element	County Data	Comments
		Identify vector-borne disease patterns in the county.	Lyme disease Spotted fever group *Rickettsiosis* Eastern equine encephalitis[6]
		Describe how most citizens obtain drinking water in the county.	Countywide water system and private wells[7]
	Weather	Describe any changes in frequency or intensity of weather issues (heat, rain, fires, snow etc.).	Summers—hot and muggy Winters—short and cold 12 months—temperatures range from 35°F to 90 °F and is rarely below 22°F or above 96°F.[8]
		Identify heat and cold-related illness and any changing patterns in the county.	This county-specific data is not found. One might find this information by accessing ER visits and Dept. of Labor statistics. Cold: hypothermia, frostbite, injuries related to icy surfaces Heat: heat stroke, heat exhaustion, dehydration
Economical Factor			
	Types of Employ-ment	Major employers Small businesses. Types of self-employment	Top 10 employers: 1.Smithfield Foods 2.Sampson County Schools 3. Prestage Farms, Inc. 4. Hog Slat Co. Inc. 5.County of Sampson 6.Sampson Regional Medical Center 7.Clinton City Schools 8. Walmart Associates Inc. 9. NC Dept. of Public Safety 10.DI & B Enterprises Inc.

---

6   North Carolina's Sampson County. (n.d.). Health Department, Sampson County Board of Health. http://www.sampsonnc.com/departments/health_department/board_of_health1.php

7   North Carolina's Sampson County. (n.d.). Water operations. http://www.sampsonnc.com/departments/public_works/water/index.php

8   WeatherSpark. (n.d.). Average weather at Sampson County Airport. https://weatherspark.com/y/146988/Average-Weather-at-Sampson-County-Airport-North-Carolina-United-States-Year-Round#Sections-BestTime

TABLE 7.1   Sampson County, North Carolina County Assessment Utilizing the
Rural Health Framework *(continued)*.

Factor	Element	County Data	Comments
			Rural areas have small businesses and people who are self-employed. The best way to gather information is by visiting the county and interviewing residents and community leaders. Inquire about engine repair shops, lawn care, carpenters, salons, other "backyard businesses."
	Charac-teristics of jobs	Hours Benefits Physical requirements Health issues/risks Full-time, part-time, seasonal	This section can be completed when on-site visits and interviews are completed. Sampson County's farmer's and farm-workers have long work hours and weeks without health benefits or paid days off. Many are part-time or sea-sonal employees. Examples of health risks are musculoskeletal strains and injury, hearing loss, depression, respi-ratory illnesses, cancer, heat-related illnesses, and HBP.
	Types of Insurance	Military	Veterans and Active Military 0.5% Compared to NC 2.1%. Compared to eastern NC counties 6.8%
		Private insurance or Employer insurance	Persons with health insurance, under the age of 64 years 81.2%. Compared to NC 87.8%. Compare to eastern NC counties 87.2%
		Uninsured	82.5% of people in county have some type of insurance. (SOTCH, 2018)
		Medicaid	Persons without health insurance, under the age of 65 years 18.8%
		Medicare	Medicaid only 26.8%. Compared to NC 18.2% Compared to eastern NC counties 21.7%
			Medicare only 5.3% Compared to NC 4.8% Compared to eastern NC counties 4.5%

TABLE 7.1   Sampson County, North Carolina County Assessment Utilizing the Rural Health Framework *(continued)*.

Factor	Element	County Data	Comments
	Economic Indicators	Average household income	This data could be calculated for locations within county or for entire county.
		Median household income	Median household income $36,742 for Sampson County.
		Poverty level	Compared to NC $48,256. Compared to the 33 county region there are only 9 counties with lower median household income.
		Net migration (increase or decrease in population)	24.2% of Sampson's population is below poverty level. Compared to NC 16.8% Compared to counties in the region 19.2% Note: People 65+ poverty rate is 13.5% Compare to NC 9.7% Counties in region 11.5%
			From 2010 to 2018 there was a 0.2% increase in the total population
	Health Care Resources[9]	Home care Hospice Health department Hospital	Liberty Home Care & Hospice Community Home Care & Hospice Sampson Home Health
		Clinics	HD is located in Clinton. Sampson County Regional Hospital is located in Clinton.
		EMS Fire/rescue departments	Clinton Medical Clinic—Primary Care Sampson Medical Group—Primary Care
		Social services programs Type of and ratio of health care professionals	Child Health Clinic—Health Department

9   Sampson County. (2019). Community health needs assessment. https://cms4.revize.com/revize/sampsoncounty/document_center/Health/2019/2019%20Sampson_County%20CHNA%20Report%20FINAL.pdf

TABLE 7.1 Sampson County, North Carolina County Assessment Utilizing the
Rural Health Framework *(continued)*.

Factor	Element	County Data	Comments
		Telehealth	There are 16 fire/EMS stations in the county.
		Farm extension service	Main location is in Clinton. There are programs for adults and children of all ages in areas such as nutrition, transportation, Medicaid, and others. Primary care physicians 4.7 per 10,000 pop. (NC 7:10,000). Dentist 1.7 per 10,000 pop. (NC 5:10,000). Psychiatrists & psychologists 0.3 per 10,000 pop (NC 3.5:10,000). OB/GYNs, family medicine, CNMs 3.7/10,000 (NC 4.2:10,000) 3HC in Clinton offers telehealth. Residents of Sampson County who have Medicaid and NCBCBS have telehealth visits covered. CES for county is located in Clinton[10] Eileen Coite, Director Danelle Graham, 4-H Youth Development Elizabeth Merrill, 4-H Program Assistant, 4–H Youth Development Genny Thompson, Extension Agent, 4–H Youth Development Paul Gonzalez, Extension Agent, Agriculture— Livestock Brad Hardison, Extension Agent, Agriculture— Horticulture James Hartsfield, Area Agent, Small Farm Management—A&T State Max Knowles, Extension Agent, Agriculture—Livestock Hunter Rhodes, Extension Agent, Agriculture—Fields Crops

---

10   North Carolina Cooperative Extension. (2020). Sampson County Center. https://sampson.ces.ncsu.edu/

TABLE 7.1   Sampson County, North Carolina County Assessment Utilizing the Rural Health Framework *(continued)*.

Factor	Element	County Data	Comments
		Sociocultural Factor	
	Health Beliefs and Value	Describe prevalence of: stoicism, independence, reliance on physical capabilities, relationships. Definition of health, use of home remedies, views of conventional health care.	Community interviews could be conducted to explore the health and beliefs held by county residents. Rural populations tend to be independent and self-reliant. They exhibit stoicism when faced with pain or illness. Being able physically to perform work duties is seen as being healthy. Health is also measured by being able to fulfill one's role in relationships or in the family. Home remedies passed down through generations are commonly used before seeking conventional therapies. Mistrust of health professionals may exist.
	Social Capital	Identify and list social networks and support systems (formal and informal) found in the county.	Formal examples of Social Capital: Clinton-Sampson Rotary Club[11] American Legion Auxiliary Unit#319 Coharie Intra-Tribal Council, Inc.[12] Schools and Fire/EMS Stations are also examples. Informal examples of social capital: friends, neighbors, coworkers, and family.
	Gathering Places	Identify and list places where people gather in the county.	Schools: Clinton City Schools—5 locations County Schools—18 locations Harrells Christian Academy Others are EMS/Fire stations, hair salons, and barber shops. Visiting the county and interviewing residents is helpful for compiling this information.

---

11   Sampson County Chamber of Commerce. (n.d.). Family, community & civic organizations. http://business.clintonsampsonchamber.org/list/ql/family-community-civic-organizations-9

12   Coharie Tribe. (2020). History. https://coharietribe.org/history/

TABLE 7.1 Sampson County, North Carolina County Assessment Utilizing the Rural Health Framework *(continued)*.

Factor	Element	County Data	Comments
	Faith-Based Organizations	Identify and list any and all churches, mosques, temples, others. List some of the health-related initiatives these FBO present.	There are 188 faith-based organizations in the county.[13] Types: Baptist Holiness Catholic Episcopal Latter Day Saints African American Episcopal Mosques Temples
	Heritage and Festivals	Identify and list festivals held in the county. List any health-related initiatives that are part of these festivals. Find and summarize information about the history and heritage of the area.	County was settled in 1700s by Scotch and Irish immigrants who farmed and logged. Coharie Tribe has a Tribal Center and is recognized by the state. There is a chief and six-member tribal council and tribal chairperson.[14] Sampson County Ag Day[15] Alive After Five Concert series Veterans Day Celebration Hubb's Farm—Field of Dreams Sampson County History Museum Day Battle of the Butts Cook-off Fall Festival Halloween Hustle Rocking for the Arts

---

13   NC Home Town Locator. (2020). Sampson County NC churches. https://northcarolina.hometownlocator.com/features/cultural,class,church,scfips,37163,startrow,76.cfm

14   Coharie Tribe. (2020). History. https://coharietribe.org/history/

15   Sampson County History Museum. (n.d.). Upcoming events. https://www.sampsonhmc.com/

TABLE 7.1   Sampson County, North Carolina County Assessment Utilizing the Rural Health Framework *(continued)*.

Factor	Element	County Data	Comments
		Demographical Factor	
	Age	Provide date regarding age distribution groups or ranges reported for county.[16]	< 5 years 6.5% <18 years 24.3% >65 years 18.3% <20 years 29.6% 20–29 years 11.8% 30–39 years 10.7% 40–49 years 13.9% 50–59 years 13.5% 60–69 years 12.1% 70–79 years 11.2% [17]
	Ethnicity	Provide data to identify ethnic groups that comprise the county. Report as a percentage of the population.	White 66.6% African Americans 26.6% Asian 0.6% Hawaiian 0.3% 2 or > races 2.3% Latino 20.6%[18]
	Gender	Provide data regarding male compared to female as a percentage of the population.	Female 50.8% Male 49.2%[19]
	Marital Status	Provide data pertaining to marital status in the county. Report as a percentage of the population.	Married 49% Never married 30% Divorced 12% Widowed 9%

16   NCIOM. (n.d.). North Carolina Health Profile—Sampson County. https://nciom.org/counties/sampson-county/

17   , 32 United States Census. (2018). QuickFacts Sampson County, North Carolina. https://www.census.gov/quickfacts/sampsoncountynorthcarolina

18

19   TownCharts. (2018). Sampson County, North Carolina Demographics Data. https://www.towncharts.com/North-Carolina/Demographics/Sampson-County-NC-Demographics-data.html

TABLE 7.1   Sampson County, North Carolina County Assessment Utilizing the
Rural Health Framework *(continued)*.

Factor	Element	County Data	Comments
	Educational level	Percentage with high school education.	HS graduate or higher, percentage of persons age 25+ years 77.7%.
		Percentage college graduates. Percentage without high school education.	Bachelor's degree or higher, percent of persons age 25+ years 12.8%
			22.3% without HS education

Support Factor

Factor	Element	County Data	Comments
	Local Governance	Local board of health[20]	Dr. Jeffery Bell, Dentist Paul Bradshaw, Chairman, Public Member Robert Butler, Engineer Linda Peterson, Public Member Charlotte Harrell, Pharmacist Linda Heath, Nurse
		County commissioners	Dr. Elizabeth Bryan, Physician Jacqueline Howard, Vice-Chair, Public Member
			Harry Parker, County Commissioner Allie Ray McCullen, Public Member Dr. Beth Turner, Veterinarian
			Clark Wooten, Chairman, District 1 **cwooten@sampsonnc.com** Jerol Kivett, District 2 **jkivett@sampsonnc.com** Sue Lee, Vice Chairperson, District 3 **slee@sampsonnc.com** Harry L. Parker, District 4 **hparker@sampsonnc.com** Thaddeus L. Godwin, District 5 **tgodwin@sampsonnc.com**[21]

20   North Carolina's Sampson County. (n.d.). Health department, Sampson County Board of Health. http://www.sampsonnc.com/departments/health_department/board_of_health1.php

21   North Carolina Sampson County. (n.d.). Sampson County Board of Commissioners. http://www.sampsonnc.com/departments/board_of_commissioners.php

TABLE 7.1 Sampson County, North Carolina County Assessment Utilizing the Rural Health Framework *(continued)*.

Factor	Element	County Data	Comments
	Federal Agencies	Centers for Disease Control (CDC)	COVID-19 prevention and testing.
		Office of Rural Health Policy (FORHP) Rural Health Research Center Program	Office of Rural Health and NCDHHS has 2 grants open: Rural Hospital Flexibility Improvement Grant 2021 Rural Health Center Capital Grant SFY 2020–2021
		Office of Rural Mental Health Research (ORMHR)	FORHP has 2 grants open: Rural Health Dissemination Program Rural Health Network Development Planning Program ORMHR contact information: Andrea Beckel-Mitchener, Ph.D. Acting Director 301-443-2847, **amitchen@mail.nih.gov**[22]
	National Programs/ Organizations	AHECs County Health Rankings CES National Organizations	Southern Regional AHEC: [23] TEACH (Teaching Excellence for a Career in Health) NC AHEC Scholars Program Youth Health Service Corp ORPCE (The Office of Regional Primary Education) Continuing Education for Health Professions NCQA Patient-Centered Medical Home Practice Support, Value-Based Care Clinical Education and Service—NC HealthConnex

22   National Institute of Mental Health. (2020). Office of Rural Mental Health Research—Overview. https://www.nimh.nih.gov/about/organization/od/office-of-rural-mental-health-research-ormhr.shtml

23   Southern Regional AHEC. (2020). Annual report 2018–2019. https://www.southernregionalahec.org/wp-content/uploads/2019/10/annual-report.pdf

TABLE 7.1   Sampson County, North Carolina County Assessment Utilizing the
Rural Health Framework *(continued)*.

Factor	Element	County Data	Comments
			Grants: FACE-IT! (Facing Addiction Through Community Empowerment and Intervention Teams) Communities Fostering Resiliency in Youth Out of 100 NC counties, Sampson County ranks 77th in terms of health outcomes. See above list of staff working out of the Sampson County Extension Office. October the Sampson Extension Service offers "Cooking Under Pressure"—healthy meals using pressure cookers. DHHS CARES NC grant
	Telehealth	Telemedicine Telepsychiatry Telepharmacy	There are 23,537 households with 79.0% having a computer and 59.6% having broadband internet. Sampson County offers Zoom meeting "Cooking Under Pressure." Statewide Telepsychiatry Program (NC-STeP) East Carolina Center for Telepsychiatry and e-Behavioral Health.[24] Telepharmacy is not found in NC.

---

24   NCDHHS. (2020). Statewide telepsychiatry program. https://www.ncdhhs.gov/divisions/office-rural-health/office-rural-health-programs/statewide-telepsychiatry-program

TABLE 7.1   Sampson County, North Carolina County Assessment Utilizing the Rural Health Framework *(continued)*.

Factor	Element	County Data	Comments
FOR GRANTS LOOK DHHS[25] HRSA[26] CMS	Health Interventions	Health centers Expanded roles: community health workers, health coaches, patient navigators	FCHCs:[27] Goshen Medical Center Tri-County Community Health Council Harrells Tri-County Community Health Council Dunn Tri-County Community Health Council Clinton Community Health Council Community Health Workers are utilized in 50 NC counties, including Sampson, to help with contact tracing during the COVID-19 pandemic.[28]

#1 Case Assessment: Immunization Rates in Rural Communities

The CDC has begun a new immunization registry program in your state as one of its pilot sites and wants to understand what factors might affect pneumonia immunization rates in rural communities. In response to this new initiative, you have been asked to work with a county health department (of a county in your area) to assess the factors affecting its immunization program for individuals over 65. To accomplish this, you need to do a focused countywide assessment.

Task 1: Complete a rural health framework community assessment grid.

Task 2: Answer these specific questions:

---

25   NCDHHS. (August 7, 2020). NCDHHS selects venders to supervise 250+ new community health workers in 50 counties with COVID-19 hot spots. https://www.ncdhhs.gov/news/press-releases/ncdhhs-selects-vendors-supervise-250-new-community-health-workers-50-counties

26   HRSA. (2020). Find funding. https://www.hrsa.gov/grants/find-funding?status=Open&bureau=642

27   DSH and FQHC Locations. (2019). [pdf]. https://files.nc.gov/ncdma/2019-Outstations-DSH-FQHC-Locations.pdf

28   NCDHHS. (August 7, 2020). NCDHHS Selects Venders to Supervise 250+ New Community Health Workers in 50 Counties with COVID-19 Hot Spots. https://www.ncdhhs.gov/news/press-releases/ncdhhs-selects-vendors-supervise-250-new-community-health-workers-50-counties

a. Since this new program is investigating rural communities specifically, does the county (a county in your area) qualify as "rural"? If so, what makes it rural? Whose definition of rural are you using? If the county (a county in your area) does not qualify, justify why and cite whose definition you are using.

b. Which elements have particular significance in addressing the project aim? For instance, age is important in determining how many people are over 65, as well as their general distribution throughout the county.

c. If a mobile van were to be used to give vaccines, where would you locate the van, and why would you choose that location

d. Are there social/cultural elements that might increase vaccine resistance among people in the county?

Task 3: Collect your findings and prepare a presentation (e.g., a PowerPoint or video presentation) to inform the county health department board of your findings.

#2 Case Assessment: Infant Mortality

Arlinda Oxendine is 7 months pregnant. She is particularly anxious about this baby since her first baby died shortly after delivery from an infection. Arlinda has attended nearly all of her prenatal visits at the (choose a county in your state) County Health Department, with only a few missed visits when she could not arrange transportation. [It is best to pick a county with a high infant mortality rate, if possible.]

Applying the Rural Heath Framework, consider the elements that comprise the demographical factor and the economical factor. Which elements could potentially impact the infant mortality rate?

#3 Case Assessment: Opioid and Substance Abuse Prevention

You are collaborating with other health professionals and community partners to address opioid addiction and substance abuse prevention in your county. The question is raised whether your area (select a county in your area) might qualify for a rural health grant.

Chose an entire county or location you believe to be rural and go to this website: https://data.hrsa.gov/tools/rural-health?tab=Address

Then enter the location into the Rural Health Grants Eligibility Analyzer. What did the analyzer tell you? Was the county or location you chose rural?

To further understand why some locations are rural and others are not, scroll to the bottom of the Rural Health Eligibility Analyzer site, and click on the national listing of eligible counties and census tracts PDF file and read the definitions of rural areas found there.

If the county you originally selected is not rural, compare the county you selected to the definitions to better understand criteria determining the rural designation. Then select an eligible county from the national listing to complete this case assessment.

One collaborative partner makes the group aware that North Carolina State Extension has a program for the prevention and reduction of opioid misuse and abuse education for youth and families in North Carolina. Go here to read about the program: https://nc4h.ces.ncsu.edu/healthy-living/empowering-youth-families-program/

As you see, this is a 4–H program and therefore serves youth from age 9 through 18. It would be important information for your group to know the number of youths that could be served by such a program in your selected rural county or location. Find the data. How many residents in your rural county are ages 9 through 18?

Lastly, identify other health resources or organizations in your county that could work together towards opioid and substance abuse prevention.

#4 Case Assessment: Pandemic—Ski Resort in Gunnison County

Gunnison County is a rural county in Colorado that is home to the Crested Butte Ski Resort. Consider how the ski resort impacts the county in regard to the COVID-19 pandemic. You might gather data/facts about the number and types of visitors to the resort. Where do they come from? What is the age range of visitors? You might also look for other businesses in the county that would attract travelers.

Learn more by exploring this website and others to gather facts/data about Gunnison County, Colorado: https://usafacts.org/visualizations/coronavirus-covid-19-spread-map/state/colorado

How many people have tested positive for COVID-19?

How many COVID-19 deaths have occurred?

What other data/facts would you collect?

Now, for comprehensive county planning apply the Rural Health Framework.

Consider the elements comprising the geographical factor and how each of the elements should be considered during a pandemic.

Gather data/facts pertaining to each of the elements comprising the geographical factor.

How might this data be utilized for health planning during a pandemic?

Consider the elements comprising the economical factor and how each of the elements should be considered during a pandemic.

Gather data/facts pertaining to each of the elements comprising the economical factor.

How might this data be utilized for health planning during a pandemic?

Consider the elements comprising the demographical factor and how each of the elements should be considered during a pandemic.

Gather data/facts pertaining to each of the elements that make up the demographical factor.

How might this data be utilized for health planning during a pandemic?

Consider the elements in the sociocultural factor and how each of the elements should be considered during a pandemic.

Gather data/facts pertaining to each of the elements of the sociocultural factor.

How might this data be utilized for health planning during a pandemic?

Consider the elements of the support factor and how each of the elements should be considered during a pandemic.

Gather data/facts pertaining to each of the elements of the support factor.

How might this data be utilized for health planning during a pandemic?

#5 Case Assessment: Journal Article Comparison

Locate an article from a peer-reviewed journal that discusses a rural health topic of your choice. As you read the article, compare the content of the article to the Rural Health Framework.

How does the article define "rural"?

Which of the 25 elements are addressed in the article?

Which of the elements are not covered in the article?

Do any of the missing elements not covered impact the perspective of the article's intent or potentially change conclusions?

Would the intent of the article be more comprehensive if all 25 elements were considered? If yes, explain how. If not, explain why not.

#6 Case Assessment: Telehealth Case Assessment

Mary Jones is a health practitioner in the county. She is interested in expanding the telehealth care programs in her clinic, especially the possibility of creating an interprofessional telehealth care team. When she approaches others, she finds that there is more interest in this delivery method than she had anticipated. You are helping her think through these findings.

Part 1:

a. Why would telehealth care be more acceptable now than in the past?
b. Who might be a good member of an interprofessional telehealth care team in a rural area?
c. What kind of telehealth care technologies should Mary consider when she talks about telehealth care, and why these particular ones (be sure to address issues of community values or beliefs)?

Part 2:

Now pick a county in your state to apply further issues within that county.

a. Describe cultural concerns that might emerge. Use the five elements of the cultural factor to inform these concerns.
b. Describe health resources as identified in the economical factor.

REFERENCES

Census of Agriculture County Profile. (2017). Sampson County North Carolina. https://www.nass.usda.gov/Publications/AgCensus/2017/Online_Resources/County_Profiles/North_Carolina/cp37163.pdf

Centers for Disease Control and Prevention. (2020). Stroke facts. https://www.cdc.gov/stroke/facts.htm

Coharie Tribe. (2020). History. https://coharietribe.org/history/

County Health Rankings & Roadmaps. (2020). North Carolina, Sampson. https://www.countyhealthrankings.org/app/north-carolina/2020/rankings/sampson/county/outcomes/overall/snapshot

DSH and FQHC Locations. (2019). https://files.nc.gov/ncdma/2019-Outstations-DSH-FQHC-Locations.pdf

HRSA. (2020). Find funding. https://www.hrsa.gov/grants/find-funding?status=Open&bureau=642

Hurricane Matthew Resilient Redevelopment Plan. (2017, May). https://files.nc.gov/rebuildnc/documents/matthew/rebuildnc_sampson_plan_combined.pdf

National Institute of Mental Health. (2020). Office of Rural Mental Health Research—overview. https://www.nimh.nih.gov/about/organization/od/office-of-rural-mental-health-research-ormhr.shtml

NC Home Town Locator. (2020). Sampson County NC churches. https://northcarolina.hometownlocator.com/features/cultural,class,church,scfips,37163,startrow,76.cfm

NCDHHS. (2020). Action pathways. https://actionpathways.ngo/

NCDHHS. (2020, August 7). NCDHHS Selects venders to supervise 250+ new community health workers in 50 counties with COVID-19 hot spots. https://www.ncdhhs.gov/news/press-releases/ncdhhs-selects-vendors-supervise-250-new-community-health-workers-50-counties

NCDHHS. (2020). Rural health grant opportunities. https://www.ncdhhs.gov/about/grant-opportunities/rural-health-grant-opportunities

NCDHHS. (2020). Statewide telepsychiatry program. https://www.ncdhhs.gov/divisions/office-rural-health/office-rural-health-programs/statewide-telepsychiatry-program

NCIOM. (n.d.). North Carolina health profile—Sampson County. https://nciom.org/counties/sampson-county/

North Carolina 2018 Traffic Crash Facts. (n.d.). https://connect.ncdot.gov/business/DMV/CrashFactsDocuments/2018%20Crash%20Facts.pdf

North Carolina Cooperative Extension. (2020). Sampson County Center. https://sampson.ces.ncsu.edu/

North Carolina Department of Health and Human Services. (2017). Vector-borne disease surveillance summary [pdf]. https://epi.dph.ncdhhs.gov/cd/vector/VBDSurvellanceSummaries2017.pdf

North Carolina Sampson County. (n.d.). Sampson County Board of Commissioners. http://www.sampsonnc.com/departments/board_of_commissioners.php

North Carolina's Sampson County. (n.d.). Health Department, Sampson County Board of Health. http://www.sampsonnc.com/departments/health_department/board_of_health1.php

North Carolina's Sampson County. (n.d.). Water operations. http://www.sampsonnc.com/departments/public_works/water/index.php#:~:text=Sampson%20County%20purchases%20its%20water,City%20of%20Dunn%20is%20maintained

Sampson County. (2019). Community health needs assessment. [pdf]. https://cms4.revize.com/revize/sampsoncounty/document_center/Health/2019/2019%20Sampson_County%20CHNA%20Report%20FINAL.pdf

Sampson County Chamber of Commerce. (n.d.). Family, community & civic organizations. http://business.clintonsampsonchamber.org/list/ql/family-community-civic-organizations-9

Sampson County Health Department. (n.d.). State of the County Health Report 2018. https://cms4.revize.com/revize/sampsoncounty/document_center/Health/2019/2018%20SOTCH%20FINAL.pdf

Sampson County Map. The Way We Lived in North Carolina. (2004). Sampson County. https://waywelivednc.com/maps/countymaps/maps/sampson.htm).

Sampson County History Museum. (n.d.). Upcoming events. https://www.sampsonhmc.com/

Southern Regional AHEC. (2020). Annual Report 2018–2019. [pdf]. https://www.southernregionalahec.org/wp-content/uploads/2019/10/annual-report.pdf

TownCharts. (2018). Sampson County, North Carolina demographics data. https://www.towncharts.com/North-Carolina/Demographics/Sampson-County-NC-Demographics-data.html

United States Census. (2018). QuickFacts Sampson County, North Carolina. https://www.census.gov/quickfacts/sampsoncountynorthcarolina

The Way We Lived in North Carolina. (2004). Sampson County. https://waywelivednc.com/maps/countymaps/maps/sampson.htm

WeatherSpark. (n.d.). Average weather at Sampson County Airport. https://weatherspark.com/y/146988/Average-Weather-at-Sampson-County-Airport-North-Carolina-United-States-Year-Round#Sections-BestTime

Figure Credits

Learning Assessment Answers

CHAPTER 1

Rural Health Terms

1. False
2. Three organizations that provide an official definition of "rural" are the Census Bureau, the Office of Management and Budget, and the Department of Agriculture & Economic Research.
3. The three dimensions of health care access that the WHO outlines are physical accessibility, financial affordability, and acceptability.
4. The nurse must pass a licensure test and be licensed in the state of practice.
5. American Nurses Association

Rural Health Concepts

1. Complex
2. Lisa Bourke and Jane Farmer
3. Five factors and 25 elements
4. The geographical factor, the sociocultural factor, the economical factor, the demographical factor, and the support factor
5. Data is collected at the level of the 25 elements.

CHAPTER 2

Location

1. Topology, county seat, county's population density, and towns/population centers
2. Any given answer that represents topographical features of the selected county. Example might be depending on the county, rivers, swamps, waterways, ocean, and islands.
3. Reasonable answer given the land feature selected as long as the solution could potentially improve health care access.

4. True
5. Social Services, courthouse, Farm Services Agency, hospital, health department, EMS, fire/rescue, sheriff office
6. Total, square miles
7. Response should include how a county with more people per square mile compared with a less densely populated county would require more funds for health care services.
8. a

Roads

1. Narrow—rural roads are narrow two-lane roads with vehicles traveling in opposite directions creating an increased likelihood of accidents and injuries.
2. No paved shoulders—rural roads are without paved shoulders, leaving no room for EMS vehicles to reach an accident. If a driver swerves off the paved surface, the absence of a paved shoulder limits a driver's ability to correct the vehicle and avoid an accident.
3. Overgrown vegetation—weeds, grasses, trees, and crops line rural roads. The vegetation can obscure a driver's ability to see obstacles and hazards, increasing the chance of an accident.
4. Curvy—rural roads are curvy, and the curves increase the likelihood losing control of a vehicle and causing an accident. The curves can also prevent a driver from seeing obstacles in the road, increasing the chance of accidents.
5. Unreliable GPS—the lack of reliable GPS signals can result in a delay in receiving care due to lack of ability to locate an accident site.
6. Damaged or missing signage—damaged or missing signage can result in a delay in receiving care due to lack of ability to locate an accident site.
7. Obstacles in the road—obstacles in the road can result in collisions and injury. Some obstacles are wildlife, farm equipment, tree limbs, and other debris.
8. Highways through rural areas can spread illnesses such as influenza in humans and avian flu in poultry and be corridors for drug transportation.
9. True
10. False

Air

1. Forest fires, concentrated animal feeding operations, dust from mining, dust from farming, abundant pollen
2. False
3. Cardiac and respiratory conditions

4. Respiratory issues such as asthma, mental health issues such as depression, migraines, diarrhea, eye irritation
5. True
6. True
7. Aerial spraying by planes flying over fields and by tractors being driven through fields
8. False
9. Asthma, rhinitis, sinusitis
10. True

Water

1. True
2. Hepatitis, giardia, campylobacter, *E.coli*, shigella, cryptosporidium, and *Salmonella*
3. True
4. Watering lawns or opening levies
5. Acid mine drainage
6. Ticks, fleas, mosquitoes, and snakes
7. Examples: mosquitoes = West Nile virus and ticks = Lyme disease
8. Place to recreate and exercise, irrigation, drinking, watering livestock, and transportation

Weather

1. True
2. Respiratory illnesses, contact dermatitis, wound infections, drownings
3. False
4. Hyperthermia
5. Dehydration, heat exhaustion, heat stroke, melanoma
6. Urban areas have malls, community centers, libraries, and businesses which act as air-conditioned places to escape the heat.
7. d.

CHAPTER 3

Income Indicators

1. Five elements that make up the economical factor: types of employment, characteristics of jobs, income indicators, health resources, and health insurance
2. d.

3. Preventative, progressed
4. c.
5. Federal government
6. Determine the household incomes for each to the households in the county. Total these numbers and divide the total by the number of households in the county.
7. False
8. True
9. False
10. Median household income, average household income, and poverty-level

Types of Employment Industries

1. True
2. a., b., c., & d.
3. Good producing industries, service producing industries, agriculture, and non-agriculture self-employed
4. Childcare, barbers/hair stylists, funeral directors, and landscapers
5. False
6. True
7. $1,000
8. True
9. Half
10. Names of major employers or employment industries are provided, but small business and self-employment are not reported. It is important to carefully review employment tables and not to overlook the self-employed and small businesses.

Job Characteristics

1. Poor pay, pay fluctuation, lack of health insurance offered by the job, few if any employee benefits, and strains on the body
2. b.
3. Fear losing job, no paid days off, lack of insurance, out-of-pocket expenses
4. True
5. Rural
6. Hours may vary resulting in pay fluctuation and job may be seasonal.
7. True
8. No paid time off, less flex hours, fewer support programs, fewer opportunities to telecommute

9. No paid days off—employees will work sick/injured to avoid missing a day's pay. Less flex hours–add to stress level when trying to balance work responsibilities and personal responsibilities. Fewer support programs—lack of wellness incentive, mental health support, or treatment for addiction. Lack of opportunity to telecommute—telecommuting can add to increased job satisfaction and sense of well-being.

10. Depression, respiratory issues, cancer, injuries, hearing loss, eye problems, exposure to temperature extremes, and musculoskeletal problems

TYPES OF INSURANCE

1. a
2. a.
3. False
4. Longer, less
5. Insurance we pay for ourselves, employee-sponsored health insurance, and government sponsored insurance
6. TRICARE
7. True
8. While there are more elderly people living in rural areas than in urban, they may not have paid into Social Security. This is a plausible explanation given the job types: temporary or seasonal employees, self-employed, or work in the home or in family-owned business.
9. False
10. True

Health Resources

1. b.
2. d.
3. a.
4. True
5. d.
6. True
7. Local economy declines, decreased tax base, delay in receiving needed health care, access to health care becomes more difficult to obtain
8. HPSA is a federal designation for shortages of primary care practitioners (medicine, PA, NP), dental, and mental health providers. Designation of a HPSA area may carry benefits in terms of available grants or funding. Professional shortage is a lack of health professionals in an area regardless of discipline (e.g., medicine, nursing, pharmacy). HPS are reported as a ratio of the population. Example 1 dentist: 10,000 population.

Thus, the term health professional shortage is a better term to describe the breadth of needs in rural communities.

9. Health education, worker safety, creation of health careers, health care workforce development, grant writing, assisting primary care providers

10. Day care centers, schools and school nurse programs, lay health care workers and local charities, parish nursing

CHAPTER 4

Beliefs and Values

1. The five elements that make up the sociocultural factor are beliefs and values, social capital, gathering places, faith-based organizations, and festivals and heritage.

2. This is a true statement.

3. Independent-minded, self-sufficient, and stoic

4. A stoic individual denies the existence of pain and would not go to see a physician until the pain became unbearable. This behavior would cause a delayed diagnosis and treatment so that an underlying disease process would be more advanced.

5. This is a false statement. The discussion of mental health issues is taboo in rural populations. If discussed at all, it would be kept in the immediate family. For this and other reasons, such as isolation, there is a high suicide rate amongst farmers.

6. This is a true statement. Alternative medicines are commonly utilized by rural populations and should be part of the health information collected.

7. Types of alternative medicine therapies are: chiropractic care, mediation, herbal medicines, massage, relaxation, and vitamins and minerals.

8. The correct answer is b. Latino agricultural workers believe in folk healers and utilize massage for pain relief.

Social Capital

1. This is a true statement.

2. Skills and resources

3. Strength and community

4. Family ties, civic involvement, religious affiliation, and residents' intersections

5. Mayor or pastors

6. These informal leaders are trusted and respected by the rural residents. Rural residents may go to these informal leaders for health advice. When planning health care

interventions these informal leaders are often identified to help customize health care to their specific county.

7. This is a true statement. Immigrants may be isolated and not benefit from social capital to bridge social and health needs. Therefore, special attention must be given to identifying subpopulations in rural communities and addressing their needs.

Gathering Places

1. This is a true statement.
2. Patrons feel safe and are more trusting in these places. Barbershops and hair salons or frequented by people they know and see with some regularity.
3. This is a true statement.
4. Fire and rescue
5. Homemakers Club and 4-H Club

Faith-Based Organizations

1. Religious
2. This is a true statement.
3. Faith
4. Teacher, counselor, arbitrator, community leader, spokesperson, and advocate
5. Mental

Heritage and Festivals

1. Heritage, festivals
2. True
3. Safe water, immunizations, weight loss, stroke identification/care, and announcements of new health services
4. Competitions
5. Educational material, curricula, resource lists, and ideas for inclusion of health-related topics in the classroom

CHAPTER 5

Age

1. Age, race/ethnic, gender, marital status, and education level
2. Children under 18 and elders 65 and older

3. In the example of children, the data could be compiled for age group 5 and under or may be grouped under the age of 18. Therefore, when reporting or comparing data we must be clear about the age of the group of children (for this example) that we are examining.

4. 25%

5. a., b., and c. are characteristics of rural children. Response d. is not characteristic, since rural children are more likely to smoke cigarettes than their urban counterparts.

6. Motor vehicle accidents, farm equipment accidents, and ATV accidents

7. True

8. Some examples include public transportation, long-term care facilities, senior centers, and businesses offering home delivery.

9. True

10. Chronic care, preventable

Race/Ethnicity

1. Health outcomes

2. All answers are correct

3. True

4. Hispanics, African Americans

5. False. African Americans have **higher** mortality outcomes than urban blacks and overall rural minorities have **higher** mortality outcomes than even rural whites, non-Hispanics.

6. True

7. Biracial

8. Language barrier, mistrust of health care system, lack of confidence in being understood, fear, legal repercussions

9. 50

10. True

Gender

1. True

2. All answers characterize the health status of rural women compared to urban women.

3. Less

4. False

5. Examples include shortages of OB-GYN practitioners, closures of rural hospitals, increased likelihood of planned deliveries, and longer distances to drive.

6. True

7. Women
8. In addition to lack of mental health providers examples include a greater culture of nondisclosure, fewer resources or education, or greater unhealthy lifestyle behaviors (e.g., alcohol consumption).
9. Responses a., b., and c. accurately characterize health behaviors of men compared to women. Men are **less likely** to engage in healthy lifestyle behaviors (e.g., engage in physical activity). This makes d. an incorrect response.
10. True

Marital Status

1. True
2. Some correct responses are healthier lifestyle (e.g., exercise more, smoke less), visit doctors on a more regular basis, have lower rates of depression, and have fewer strokes and heart attacks.
3. True
4. Data shows 65% of persons 25 and older with college degree were married compared to 50% of persons with no education beyond high school.
5. The statement is false as stated. The following is a true statement: Rural children growing up in poor households have rates **higher** than the national average to marry and to marry at a younger age and **higher** than their urban counterparts in same income households.
6. True

Education Level

1. Improved, longer, greater
2. True
3. False
4. Population density is calculated by dividing the total population by the square miles. Without considering population density, the data could be misleading because there are more persons overall living in urban/suburban areas than in rural areas.
5. Lower, lower
6. False
7. Workforce, new skill

CHAPTER 6

Local Governance

1. Local governance, federal agencies, national programs/organizations, telehealth, health interventions
2. This is a true statement.
3. Oversight of the health department could include the following:
   - hiring and evaluation of the public health director
   - adopting/revising public health rules/regulations
   - assessing community health needs
   - assisting with workforce development
   - serving as liaison with other local entities or state agencies
   - serving as a community voice in the design/implementation of public health programs

4. This is a false statement. County commissioners are elected officials by voters in the county.
5. Examples of how county commissioners serve their county:

   - Listen to residents and represent the concerns of residents at meetings and to the appropriate officials.
   - Attend community events and festivals.
   - Help attract businesses to rural areas.
   - Educate and communicate upcoming county changes to residents.

Federal Agencies

1. The four federal agencies discussed in this section are the Centers for Disease Control (CDC), the Federal Office of Rural Health Policy (FORHP), the Rural Health Research Center Program, and the Office of Rural Mental Health Research (ORMHR).
2. COPD, cancer, suicide, antibiotic usage, vaccination
3. These programs are the Community Based Division (CBD), the Hospital State Division (HSD), the Office for the Advancement of Telehealth (OAT), and the Policy Research Division (PRD).
4. Health care and population health
5. The ORMHR is mandated by Congress to coordinate the research activities for the Department of Health and Human Services related to the mental health of residents

of rural areas, and to coordinate and synergize Health and Human Services activities with critical related activities of public and nonprofit entities.

National Programs/Organizations

1. Area Health Education Centers, County Health Rankings, Cooperative Extension Service, National Rural Health Association
2. Suggestions for correct response:

   a. AHEC—recruit, train, and retain health professions for underserved populations; provide clinical sites for students; provide pipeline for rural students to enter health professions; offer housing to students on location; provide practice management services
   b. County Health Rankings—provide annual data elements; provide county-level data; present comparative data; provide nutrition programs; provide youth programs
   c. CES—enhance agricultural and technical education; conducts application research; partner with land-grant universities; maintain research stations; extension agents are educators working directly with county residents
   d. NRHA—provide leadership with addressing rural health issues; advocate; educate; conduct research; publish papers; hold conferences; maintain state-level associations

3. This is a false statement. AHEC is a public or nonprofit organization.
4. c. Annually
5. The Smith-Lever Act of 1914

Telehealth

1. Telemedicine, telepsychiatry, telepharmacy
2. This is a true statement.
3. This state is false. Telehealth can allow more access to health providers and particularly specialist. Collaboration of providers is made easier through telehealth.
4. Video conferencing, telephone, email, remote monitoring
5. East Carolina

Health Interventions

1. Rural health centers and expanded roles
2. Rural health centers
3. Expanded roles
4. Community-based
5. Community health worker, health coach, patient navigator, community paramedic

About the Authors

MARIA C. CLAY

Maria is an educator, having received a master's degree in education from East Carolina University and a doctorate in education from the University of North Carolina at Chapel Hill. She had the good fortune to serve as Co-PI for the Quentin N. Burdick Program for Rural Interdisciplinary Training, which allowed her to learn firsthand the issues and challenges in rural health. To sustain this knowledge, she co-developed the Interdisciplinary Rural Health Education undergraduate and graduate coursework and has enjoyed teaching these courses to hundreds of students. Maria's interest in the social determinants of health and her subsequent training in bioethics ultimately led her to her current roles of chair of the Department of Bioethics and Interdisciplinary Studies in the Brody School of Medicine and director of the Office of Clinical Skills Assessment and Education at East Carolina University. In all these endeavors she has been fortunate to work with creative, caring, and committed colleagues, community leaders, and students. For that she is most grateful.

REBECCA W. LEWIS

Rebecca has spent her life living and working in rural eastern North Carolina. She was born and raised on a family farm and is presently immersed in family farming life. Rebecca's professional career began as a bachelor's degree-prepared nurse at a rural hospital. She later became the chief nurse executive of an acute care rural hospital. While in her hospital leadership role, she attended the University of North Carolina Chapel Hill to earn a master's degree in public health with a focus in health policy and administration. Later, while teaching associate degree nursing students and pursuing a master's degree in nursing with an emphasis in education at East Carolina University, she was introduced to the North Carolina Agromedicine Institute. She worked as the Institute's strategic planning coordinator, developing their 5-year strategic plan and furthering their mission of promoting the health and safety of agricultural populations. She co-teaches an online interdisciplinary rural health course for undergraduate students at East Carolina University.

9 781516 586202